SOLVED: THE RIDDLE OF WEIGHT LOSS

A doctor's nutritional and medical breakthrough
helps you understand the underlying causes of excess weight
and how your body chemistry can work for you.

SOLVED:

THE RIDDLE
OF WEIGHT LOSS

STEPHEN LANGER, M.D.
WITH JAMES F. SCHEER

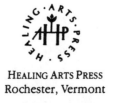

HEALING ARTS PRESS
Rochester, Vermont

Healing Arts Press
One Park Street
Rochester, Vermont 05767
Web Site: http://www.gotoit.com

Note to the reader: This book is intended as an informational guide. The remedies,
approaches, and techniques described herein are meant to supplement, and not to be
a substitute for, professional medical care or treatment. They should not be used to
treat a serious ailment without prior consultation with a qualified healthcare professional.

Library of Congress Cataloging-in-Publication Data

Langer, Stephen E.
    [How to win at weight loss]
    Solved—the riddle of weight loss / Stephen Langer, with James F. Scheer.
       p. cm.
    Originally published under the title: How to win at weight loss.
    Bibliography: p.
    Includes index.
    ISBN 0-89281-296-6
    ISBN 978-0-89281-296-7
    1. Obesity—Etiology. 2. Reducing. 3. Holistic medicine.
  I. Scheer, James F. II. Title.
  RC628.L26 1989
  613.2'5–dc20   89–7572
                                                CIP

Printed and bound in the United States

10 9 8 7 6 5

Healing Arts Press is a division of Inner Traditions International

Distributed to the book trade in Canada by Publishers Group West (PGW), Toronto,
Ontario

Distributed to the health food trade in Canada by Alive Books, Toronto and
Vancouver

CONTENTS

In the field of weight loss, new information comes to light at such a rapid rate that it is impossible for any book on the subject to include all the latest findings. If you would like to have the most current information on any of the subjects covered in this book, send a self-addressed, stamped, business envelope to:

Weight Loss and Nutrition Update
P.O. Box 1549
Lafayette, CA 94549-1549

To Debbie with love

PREFACE

Your Bill of Rights for Wellness and Weight Loss

In the land of the right-handed, the left-handed are unorthodox. The word *unorthodox* does not mean that left-handers can't get the job done—not at all. *Solved: The Riddle of Weight Loss* may be regarded by the right-handed medical profession as a left-handed approach because it leans heavily on optimum nutrition.

I am not troubled by this, because doctors usually favor medicine over applied clinical nutrition in coping with health problems. Further, the weight loss program presented in this book works, and that is what is important.

Admittedly, there is controversy about clinical nutrition, and its role in health maintenance and the treatment of disease, but this does not negate its critical role in both of these areas.

The medical profession has made some interesting detours in its healing methods since Hippocrates, the father of modern medicine, who believed in achieving and maintaining optimal health through reasonable work, lots of rest, sensible eating, and adequate sleep and recreation.

Hippocrates accepted the psychosomatic nature of human beings. He maintained that our regimen, including diet, should be the first line of attack on illness. He stated that the physician's responsibility was to assist nature, which did the curing. Second came medicine. Then, if these two failed, he turned to surgery, when indicated.

My approach is a modified Hippocratic one in which I cooperate with the body-mind to bring about health and, especially, in this book, weight loss by natural methods that do not penalize health, well-being, and longevity.

Today, natural healing and clinical nutrition are held in great disdain by organized medicine. Whole books have been written about the underlying reasons for this attitude: economic, political, and vested interests.

The standard medical modus operandi is called allopathy, the treatment of disease by remedies that bring about effects different from or opposite to those produced by the disease. This is a mechanistic approach in which symptoms are scrupulously catalogued into syndromes and disease states. No expense is spared by manufacturers of medical instrumentation and makers of drugs for medical diagnosis and treatment to rid the body of its illness.

Drug companies have only limited patent protection for products that are years in the making and often cost fortunes to produce. Quick profits have to be realized to justify their investment of time, personnel, and capital.

As a result, both physician and the media are constantly bombarded with propaganda that this drug or piece of equipment is the hoped-for breakthrough—which, in fact, it is, until the next breakthrough comes along.

Nutrients and natural products have no place in this picture, because they are unpatentable and, therefore, can never justify the research and development costs to prove they are effective.

Who would want to do a million-dollar, double-blind, crossover study to prove that vitamin C knocks out virus better than any drug on the market or has the potential of going a long way to treat such modern scourges as AIDS and cancer?

The simple answer is no one would. Linus Pauling, twice a Nobel laureate, has had numerous grant proposals to study clinical effects of vitamin C turned down.

A physician friend of mine lost his medical privileges at a local hospital because he dared to challenge the medical staff by adding vitamin C to the intravenous solutions of cancer patients (whom he was also treating with more traditional methods). He was branded a quack.

Doctors in a group called the American Academy of Medical Preventics, who use an I.V. solution of an FDA-approved drug (Di Sodium EDTA) to remove hardening of the arteries, have been viciously harassed for the past fifteen years.

The simple fact is that no one will spend a cent on medical research that can't be protected or patented.

Unfortunately, this rather broad picture is only part of the story. Not only are natural healing agents not tested, they are not tolerated.

The reason? Consider a scenario in which you're the chief executive of a company that manufactures a cold medicine. Out of nowhere comes a prominent scientist who says that two cents' worth of vitamin C can knock out a common cold in one to three days.

What would your response be? Right! You would label his assertion as cultish quackery and the scientist as a madman or charlatan for not playing the game correctly, not carrying out massive, double-blind crossover studies that have been published in a peer-review journal.

Because of the power of the mass media, the scientist's name and reputation probably would be subjected to public ridicule, adding to the confusion most of us have about who's right, who's telling the truth, and who's in it only for money.

Whatever happened to the old health dictum, "First, do no harm"? If a scientist or clinician with a good reputation claims a nontoxic, noninvasive approach to a clinical state or illness that otherwise would be treated with powerful drugs, isn't it worthwhile to give it a try—particularly if the condition is not life threatening?

As it is, powerful drugs are used in treatment with non-therapeutic poison that is just as powerful. Their negative aspects are euphemistically called side effects. The other option in traditional medicine is irreversible surgery.

Homeopathy and clinical nutrition are not pursued in depth in medical schools; doctors, fearing the medical and legal consequences, justifiably shy away from anything not in the mainstream. In addition, it makes me sad to report that many doctors are "down on" what they're not "up on" and tend to classify anyone making claims in this area as a food faddist or health fanatic.

This is not to say that unscrupulous claims are not made in this and many other fields to con the gullible. They are—but few, if any, of us ever have really stopped to think just who these gullible people are who reach for the stars every time a new health claim is made.

Many of them are those who are not cured by traditional means—individuals who fall between the cracks of the medical system, people who are told, "It's all in your head. Go home and learn to live with it," or, "You're under stress, burned out. See a psychiatrist."

A high percentage of these medical rejects are suffering from real organic and biochemical problems that our medical system is not equipped to deal with, and so they are given up as hopeless misfits.

If any of them should find relief with a medical alternative, it just corroborates the original diagnosis of hypochondriasis or neurosis since any alternatives to the system don't work "or we'd be using them."

My purpose here is not to write an exposé on the shortcomings of allopathic medicine.

Instead, I accent the positive, the benefits with virtually no risk of the nutritional approach, as stated in testimony by Bernard Rimland, Ph.D. on *Vitamin Safety vs Drugs* before a United States Senate committee on Nutrition and Human Needs (95th Congress, First Session):

". . . Vitamins are immeasurably safer than drugs which are sometimes given to children. A recent report has shown, for example, a relationship between amphetamines and the later occurrence of Hodgkins disease . . ."

Now is the time for you to make a choice. *No one* else cares as much about you as you, and you owe it to yourself to become as knowledgeable about your health as you possibly can.

By all means, make sure you capitalize on all the *best* technologies medicine has to offer, but use this information as only one of many tools to further your goal of good health as you reduce weight.

Every weight-loss technique, method, and approach in *Solved: The Riddle of Weight Loss* has been used for decades by medical doctors, pioneers who have risked their reputations and livelihoods to serve humankind, staying with the injunction, "First, do no harm." However, *never before have they been presented in one book!*

What I am stressing here is that you have your own Bill of Rights, your freedom of choice among allopathic medicine, or alternatives, or a combination. You pay the bill. You can buy what you like.

Dr. Benjamin Rush, a signer of the Declaration of Independence said it better than I possibly could. Dr. Rush had proposed that health freedom be made a part of the Bill of Rights, a guaranteed right under the United States Constitution. His recommendation didn't receive enough votes to pass, only because others felt that the existing Bill of Rights provided for guaranteed health freedom.

Does it?

Rush wrote:

"The Constitution of this republic should make provision for healing freedom. To restrict the art of healing to one class of men and deny equal privileges to others will constitute the Bastille of medical science. Such restrictions are fragments of monarchy, and have no place in a republic."

ACKNOWLEDGMENTS

If it were not for my patients who lost unwanted poundage in many unusual ways, I would not be in a position to acknowledge the help of anyone in writing this book.

There would have been no book. It is that simple. If it were not for them, I would have had no weight loss program to share with you.

If it were not for colleagues in the medical profession who encouraged me—with comments such as, "This is the first new and sound system for losing weight in a generation"—I would not have launched this book.

With that said, let me give my heartfelt thanks, first, to my collaborator, James F. Scheer, health/nutrition editor/writer, who gave me the benefit of decades of knowledge in this field and the highest quality writing skills to make this book a reality.

Let me also offer heartfelt thanks to Carolyn Scheer, Jim's wife, whose dedicated research work melded with Jim's efforts to bring this book about. I also acknowledge Carolyn's editing and typing of this manuscript under the most adverse circumstances. The Scheers are some kind of team!

I also acknowledge the time, consideration, and generous cooperation given to me and my collaborator by the following people:

Grant Gwinup, M.D., professor and chairman of endocrinology and metabolism at the University of California, Irvine; Cary Cooper, Ph.D., professor of organizational psychology at the University of Manchester (England) Institute of Science and

Technology, who supplied a list of the most stressful occupations; Edward R. Pinckney, M.D., and Cathey Pinckney, his wife, of Beverly Hills, California, for their unstinting help; Willem Khoe, M.D., Ph.D., and his wife, Judy, of Las Vegas, Nevada, who make it a daily practice to help others; and James Braly, M.D., president of Optimum Health Laboratories in Encino, California, for pertinent information on food sensitivities and allergies.

Special thanks go to William Crook, M.D., of Jackson, Tennessee, and Alice Spragins, of his staff, for gracious cooperation in permitting use of the Candida albicans questionnaire in our book.

Our thanks also go to David W. Eggleston, D.D.S., of Newport Beach, California, for permitting us to use the fruit of his research on amalgam dental fillings in the chapter *Heavy Metals, Heavy People*.

We extend our gratitude to Bill Francis, executive director of the Natural Food Associates, Inc., of Atlanta, Texas, for letting us use material from *Natural Food and Farming Digest* and for generous advice.

We salute Barbara Bassett, editor/publisher of *Bestways*, for her special methods of reducing fat in the diet.

Last and, by far, not least, we thank the editorial staff of Thorsons Publishers, Inc., for applying those invaluable final touches to this manuscript to make it the kind of book that Jim Scheer and I had hoped it would be.

Thank you, everybody!

Stephen E. Langer, M.D.

1 | Unexpected Solutions

Are you weary of the typical scenario—winning an occasional battle against overweight and losing the war?

Are you disillusioned about countless "miracle" diets and weight-reduction plans that have proved to be less than miraculous?

Then you've probably said, "*Enough!* It's time to get help."

So you signed up for one of the franchised weight-loss programs that offer a multi-pronged approach, including, but not limited to: (1) support groups (often comforting); (2) frequent weigh-ins to keep you motivated; (3) easy-to-follow diets; (4) prepackaged foods to eliminate calorie-counting and guesswork; and (5) aerobic exercise routes.

Like other earnest persons, you dedicated hard effort, much time, and much money to the cause. At first, pounds melted off, and your bathroom scale was a supportive friend. Then the weight loss slowed down, and eventually stopped; you gained again, and the bathroom scale turned into a mocking enemy. Soon you surrendered to old habits, and surplus poundage scored another victory.

If the above script even comes close to your weight-loss history, this book is for you. It was written to offer an alternative weight loss program that shows you why you haven't been able to lose weight and keep it off and, equally important, how you can.

This system really works—"works wonders," say my patients. It offers new hope and a new plan for you and other disappointed or disillusioned dieters. In my Berkeley, California, preventive-medicine practice, I chanced upon a simple yet effective weight-loss system based on solid research. This has withstood seven years of extensive testing.

WEIGHT-LOSS WITHOUT REALLY TRYING

Actually, I was shown the reality and validity of this system by overweight patients who came to me to be treated for other conditions and, in the process, lost appreciable weight without even trying. The gist of it deserves to stand tall in a paragraph by itself:

BEFORE YOU CAN LOSE WEIGHT PERMANENTLY ON ANY PROGRAM, YOU MUST ELIMINATE THE MOST COMMON, USUALLY UNDETECTED MEDICAL CAUSES FOR OVERWEIGHT AND OBESITY.

Contrary to popular opinion, there is not just a single cause for overweight. Therefore, there is no single solution, despite what books, magazine articles, and news stories claim.

Several cases from my medical files will demonstrate why you need your own individual weight-reduction program. So will many others in chapters to come.

CASE OF THE MISSING POUNDS

Jo Anne, an attractive, somewhat heavyset thirty-year-old stockbroker, suffered from bone-chilling coldness and dragging fatigue. Only the continuous drinking of black coffee hyped her through office hours.

An easy-to-administer, no-cost home test—to be described later—revealed Jo Anne's extremely low body temperature, which, along with other symptoms and her medical history, showed that she was hypothyroid, that her thyroid gland output of hormones was subnormal.

I prescribed a half grain of natural desiccated thyroid daily, adding another half grain during the next two weeks. Her temperature rose along with her energy level, and she achieved a bonus value without changing her diet. She lost twenty-three pounds—weight that stayed off—and could fit neatly into clothes she felt she would never again wear.

Diane, a bright, thirtyish homemaker, had numerous disquieting symptoms: constipation, frequent depression, and numerous respiratory infections, which her former doctor had treated with a long series of antibiotics.

In the wake of these treatments, Diane had become jittery and exhausted. She had indulged in sweets—seductive pastries, candy, and ice cream—and had rapidly added ten pounds of new padding to go with her existing excess weight.

Her previous medical treatment and symptoms led me to believe she was suffering from Candida albicans, a debilitating yeast infection which is far more prevalent than many physicians and patients are aware.

I treated her without antibiotics (by a simple yet effective method to be fully described in the upcoming chapter on Candida albicans, *The Yeast Crisis and Overweight.*) This includes omission from the diet of certain refined carbohydrate foods. Diane's infection gradually disappeared. Then, slowly, her excess weight melted away—twenty-seven pounds.

Diane exulted because her husband, the mirror, and her better fitting wardrobe said complimentary things about her new figure.

"And I didn't even have to go through the agony of dieting," she told me.

STRESS CAN ADD WEIGHT

Lynda, a young, plump newspaper reporter, came to me with a problem that challenged solution.

"Dr. Langer, my nerves are jangled, and every previous doctor recommended that I take it easy and stay on tranquilizers," she said. "I can't function in my job when I'm doped up like a zombie. Another thing, my weight is getting out of hand. I'm a butterball."

After a lengthy interview to dig to the root of her ailment, I hit a nerve in bluntly asking what in her job stressed her most.

She thought for an instant, then leveled with me.

"Doctor, I hate interviewing people who don't want to talk. I'm always afraid of coming away without a story, being chewed out by my editor, or even being fired."

"Maybe you should work at something less stressful."

"No, Doctor; I love writing and editing."

My experience in the media—writing medical articles and columns for newspapers, magazines, and a newspaper syndicate—led me to advise:

"Why don't you just ask for a transfer to copy editing or feature writing?"

Lynda nodded.

"I have."

Lynda's case has a happy ending. The newspaper started a weekly medical-nutrition section. She was made its assistant editor, and was relieved from the stress of interviewing difficult individuals and of daily deadlines.

All I had done for her was listen sympathetically, advise her, cut out all medical tranquilizers, and put her on nature's tranquilizers: a daily vitamin B-complex tablet containing 100 mg of the following fractions: B-1, B-2, B-6, B-12 (100 mcg); niacinamide, folic acid (400 mcg); pantothenic acid, biotin (100 mcg); choline, inositol and para-amino benzoic acid, plus 1,200 mg of easily assimilable oyster-shell calcium, 600 mg of magnesium, and 200 mg of vitamin D.

It was not the same Lynda who visited my office two months later. Calm and self-assertive, she was ecstatic about her new job—but, most of all, about losing thirty-one pounds.

"Dr. Langer, I don't understand my dramatic weight loss," she said. "I'm still eating the same things."

"Under stress, you eat more food and more often than you are aware, Lynda. Even more important, the stressed body produces excess endorphins, which stimulate the appetite for fattening foods."

SLEUTHING PAYS OFF

Another patient, thirty-eight-year-old Russ, was a somewhat overweight, middle-management electronics company executive. He had several problems: frequent debilitating migraine headaches (often on one side of the head), accompanying nausea, and occasional visual disorders. His history also told of binge eating, usually right after a meal.

Distressed, Russ asked, "Do you suppose I have a brain tumor, Doctor?"

"Not very likely. You may have an allergy to one or more foods."

On the verge of referring him to a clinical ecologist in the same building, I asked another question and then was hooked on the case.

"Do you have binges at the same time of day?"

"Usually in the morning, right after breakfast. Then I rush over to the plant cafeteria and have another meal—most often the same as I had had earlier."

"Do you frequently eat the same breakfast?"

"On weekdays."

"Do you usually get your migraines after weekday breakfasts?"

Somewhat surprised, he replied, "Come to think of it, yes!"

It turned out that at his apartment he habitually prepared eggs and bacon, and added a Danish roll or two and coffee with cream.

"Do you have the same breakfast when you eat out and with the same results?"

"Yes."

"What breakfast do you eat on weekends?"

"Usually, a small steak, hash browns, and pumpernickel toast. Also coffee with cream."

"Do you binge after a weekend breakfast?"

"Rarely."

Now the sleuthing became interesting.

Obviously, he was allergic to something in his weekday

breakfasts. Wheat, eggs, and milk are some of the most common documented allergens for causing migraine headaches.

"Now, Russ, do you ever eat the weekday foods for breakfast on weekends?"

"Now and then."

"Think back carefully. Did you binge after that kind of breakfast on a weekend?"

After some deliberation, he replied, "No."

"Then there's got to be a cause in your work environment."

After much probing, I learned that Russ arrived at the plant as early as 6:00 or 6:30 a.m. to deal with paperwork before the phones came alive.

"Do you react physically to anything in that environment?"

"When I first come in, I notice that my eyes sometimes water or I sneeze."

After a long question-and-answer session, we narrowed it down. Each morning shortly before Russ arrived at the plant, a maintenance man polished the corridors' vinyl flooring with a special chemical formula.

As many clinical ecologists have discovered, such work-environment pollutants—also certain insecticides, toilet-bowl cleaners, and bathroom deodorizers—trigger binge eating in some individuals.

Later tests revealed that Russ was allergic to the wheat in his Danish rolls and to eggs—the very foods he repeated after the environmental allergy set off his need to eat again.

Russ eliminated his food allergens, requisitioned an air purifier for his office, and was delivered from migraines, binge eating, and—totally, unexpectedly—from twenty-three unnecessary pounds.

NO LIFE-DISRUPTING DIETARY CHANGES

These cases are not isolated. I have many more of a similar nature in my files covering individuals who lost from 20 to 100 pounds without making life-disrupting dietary changes. My point is that, although calories do count, overweight can originate from many causes, some not generally recognized. After hypothyroidism, Candida albicans, stress, food and environmental allergies, hypoglycemia (low blood sugar), depleted adrenal glands, heavy-metals intoxication, a stressed system, and subclinical nutrition, there's still poor digestion, transport assimilation, and excretion.

In chapters to come, you will learn how to find out whether some of these usually unsuspected contributors to overweight and obesity are at the root of your problem. Equally important, you will be shown how to eliminate them. This system's purpose is to reveal why you can't lose weight for good, and to show you how you can. There's also a wealth of new, revealing information coming up on diet and exercise and how to make them work most efficiently for you.

The promise that all you must do to lose weight is take in fewer calories than you burn is a gross oversimplification. That is why most weight-loss programs don't work for most persons. This system is the first program that takes into consideration your individuality. One of its major goals is to upgrade your physical condition before recommending fewer calories and extensive exercise. Many weight-loss regimens have a high failure rate because many individuals are in too poor physical condition to endure spartan, low-calorie diets or to exercise.

Temporary weight loss—off again, on again—is an exquisite torture to persons who long to be thin. Instead of making half-hearted efforts, why not commit yourself to complete body-mind realignment that will allow you to shed permanently the pounds you can do without—a program that will bring desired results without the punishment of starvation diets or grueling marathons?

Thanks to my patients, I am able to share with you a system which will pinpoint *why* you are overweight, and *why* you stay that way. You will learn how to examine your specific physical condition, environment, and belief system (how you rate in your own eyes)—every major element of your daily life that delays, detours, or derails your weight-loss achievement.

At the same time, this book offers a weight-loss program— no, a *revolution*—based on appetizing and nutrition-rich foods, which will build bouncy good health and super-energy.

An extravagant promise?

Try the chapters to come and see for yourself.

2 | A Common Cause

A neophyte mountain climber could scale Mount Everest easier than an overweight person with hypothyroidism could lose significant poundage without correcting this medical condition.

Although easily manageable, hypothyroidism is not usually treated because few individuals even realize they have it. You could be among them.

In our previous book, *Solved: The Riddle of Illness* (Keats Publishing, Inc., 1984), health editor/writer James F. Scheer and I cited the fact that some 40 percent of the population is suffering from hypothyroidism because this disorder often escapes detection by conventional blood tests (the most common procedure used).

Dr. Gerald S. Levey, an endocrinologist and chief of medicine at the University of Pittsburgh School of Medicine, adds a hearty "Amen" in a paper, "Hypothyroidism: A Treacherous Masquerader," in *Acute Care Medicine*. His findings show that hypothyroidism often is so subtle a disease that physicians can easily misinterpret symptoms.[1]

According to Dr. Levey, diagnosing hypothyroidism on the basis of symptoms alone is complicated by the fact that its many symptoms are not generally associated with hypothyroidism: blood abnormalities (easy bruising and minor bleeding, copious blood flow in menstruation, as well as anemia); excessive blood uric acid; persistent low back pain; severe muscle cramps, especially at night; joint stiffness (mild arthritis); and a decrease in heart contractility. These disorders can be improved or relieved by thyroid hormone therapy, he writes.

Levey believes traditional testing of thyroid function may not be worth the money, in that many factors distort its results— among them, drugs and certain systemic states.

A DO-IT-YOURSELF TEST WORKS

In contrast, the Barnes Basal Temperature Test is accurate, and you can perform it yourself with a common oral thermometer. Its originator, Broda O. Barnes, M.D., Ph.D., an international authority on the thyroid, spent some forty-four years studying all aspects of this gland in university research laboratories and in his medical practice. He published more than one hundred papers on this subject in medical journals here and abroad.

Early in his career, Dr. Barnes discovered the basis for his test in almost two generations of medical literature: *a common denominator in hypothyroidism is subnormal temperature.* When metabolism is low, body temperature also is low. Every hypothyroid patient who came to him for treatment verified his finding.

In his book, *Hypothyroidism: The Unsuspected Illness*,[2] Barnes described his experiments with 1,000 college students, which established the correlation of low body temperature and hypothyroidism. His test was listed in the *Physician's Desk Reference* (PDR) for many years.

Many physicians in the United States and abroad—the number grows each month—use this test in preference to blood tests, which are specific for hypothyroidism but not sensitive enough. These medical doctors—I among them—have found that even subclinical hypothyroidism as small as a fraction of a degree below normal can bring on one or more symptoms, including a tendency to add weight.

The first step in Dr. Langer's weight-loss program is taking the Barnes Basal Temperature Test to rule out hypothyroidism or to treat it if it exists. Here's how!

THE ABC'S

On the night before the test, shake down an oral thermometer and leave it on your bedside table. The very moment you wake up after a good night's sleep—no alcohol the night before, please—stay in bed and place the thermometer firmly in the armpit, leaving it there for ten minutes. (*Do not take your temperature by mouth!* Although mouth and armpit temperatures are identical under ideal circumstances, sore throats, colds, and sinusitis raise oral temperature, giving a false reading.)

If your reading is lower than 97.8—normal resting temperature—even if just a fraction below, you are very likely hypothyroid. Repeat the process on the next morning. *If you are a woman of child-bearing years, perform the test on only the second and third days of menstruation.*

CHECK OUT THESE SYMPTOMS

The following are the most common hypothyroidism symptoms that my patients have experienced in order of their greatest frequency:

1. Fatigue.
2. Feeling cold, particularly in the hands and feet.
3. Weight gain or inability to lose weight, despite constant attempts at dieting.
4. Lethargy.
5. Dry, coarse skin.
6. Swelling eyelids.
7. Coarse hair.
8. Pale skin.
9. Enlarged heart.
10. Faulty memory.
11. Constipation.
12. Hair loss.

13. Labored, difficult breathing.

14. Swelling feet.

15. Hoarseness.

16. Nervousness.

17. Depression.

18. Menstrual problems (excessive bleeding, painful menstruation, irregular periods, scanty flow or cessation of menstruation before the right age [amenorrhea]).

19. Loss of sexual desire and enjoyment of sex (low libido).

20. Impotence.

21. Heart palpitation.

22. Emotional instability.

23. Brittle nails.

24. Muscle weakness, pain.

25. Pain in joints.

26. Poor concentration and memory.

27. Anemia.

28. Atherosclerosis.

29. High cholesterol levels.

YOUR FAMILY MEDICAL HISTORY

If you have two or more of the first five symptoms and/or six or more of the remaining twenty-five symptoms, there's good reason to check your medical history. But first, you will need some information on the world's goiter belts—areas where the soil is deficient in iodine, the thyroid gland's nutritional constituent.

Before pinpointing them, I should tell you that, although your thyroid gland requires only a minute amount of iodine—100–200 micrograms or millionths of a gram per day—to remain well nourished, soils of goiter belts supply only about one-seventh the amount needed.

1. Were you or your parents born in a mountainous or inland region—the valley of the St. Lawrence River (United States or Canada), the Appalachian Mountains, the Great Lakes basin or westward through Minnesota, South Dakota, Montana, Wyoming (also adjoining areas in Canada), the Rocky Mountains on into the Northwest (areas of Oregon, Washington, and British Columbia); in Europe's Alps, Carpathian, or Pyrenees mountains; Asia's Himalaya Mountains or South America's Andes Mountains? Did you or your parents live in any of these regions for twenty years or more?

2. Have you or has either of your parents or any immediate family member ever had a goiter?

3. Have you or has either of your parents or any immediate family member suffered from thyroiditis (inflammation of the thyroid gland)?

If your Barnes Basal Temperature Test shows subnormal temperature, if you have two or more of the most frequently experienced symptoms (the first five) and/or six or more of the latter symptoms, and if you can answer "yes" to any of the medical history questions, you are most likely hypothyroid.

FORGET THE PATIENT, CONSIDER THE TEST

Despite the validity of this three-phase approach, you may have some difficulty convincing your doctor that you are hypothyroid, particularly if his or her approach is conventional. This is because most doctors place total reliance on the laboratory tests that measure blood levels of thyroid hormones. These tests are specific for thyroid diagnosis but not nearly sensitive enough to pick up the overwhelming number of people who are suffering from hypothyroidism.

One of my disillusioned physician friends sums up the situation thus:

"These doctors keep lab test results and throw out the patients."

Edward R. Pinckney, M.D., former associate editor of the *Journal of the American Medical Association*, wrote a revealing article for the *Archives of Internal Medicine*, showing well-documented inaccuracies of laboratory tests as disclosed by Food and Drug Administration investigations and by the fact that the American College of Physicians evaluated the usefulness of medical testing and found fifty common tests to be "of no proven value, unreliable or obsolete."[3]

Dr. Pinckney favors comparing medical test results with the physician's clinical judgment. "If the doctor relies solely on laboratory tests, what good are his or her training and experience?"

In a Mayo Clinic study, Drs. Joseph L. Scott Jr. and Elizabeth Mussey discovered that patients could be evaluated as mildly hypothyroid by one physician and normal by another, if diagnosis is based on a single test or office interview.[4]

THYROID HORMONES: TREMENDOUS TRIFLES

Why is thyroid function so important to good health and to weight control?

For several reasons. Every cell in your body requires three things, without which life would not be possible: oxygen, nutrients, and thyroid hormones.

The thyroid is the largest endocrine gland in the body. It secretes just one teaspoon of hormones each year—in infinitesimal increments as needed. However, if your body is slightly shortchanged of this precious substance, you are in big trouble.

This small amount of hormones, a tremendous trifle, controls the metabolic working of each of the trillions of cells that add up to become you, from your hair follicles to your toenails.

Think of the thyroid hormone as a cellular carburetor. If your carburetor is set too low, your biochemical motor won't produce the necessary energy for peak efficiency. You feel washed out, your hands and feet may be cold, and you can't lose weight, no matter how desperately you try. (This is not to say that *all* hypothyroids are overweight. Dr. Barnes found that some 39 percent are normal in weight. My statistics on patients are similar.)

Let's extend the carburetor analogy to common combustion to clarify the subject further. Have you ever tried to build a fire with damp logs? You get very little heat and lots of smoke.

That's what happens in your cells if you're hypothyroid. The cells are sluggish and underfunctioning. The most common consequences in your body are poor blood circulation, poor assimilation of nutrients, and inability to eliminate body wastes efficiently.

We have already named almost thirty of the most common symptoms of hypothyroidism. However, there are more than 100. Unfortunately, many of them are tragically mistaken for other serious medical conditions if low thyroid is not first ruled out.

BORN TIRED

The most common, telltale complaint to watch for in low thyroid function is fatigue—mild to unbearable. No amount of sleep eliminates it. People who have it seem to have been born tired and become even more so with passing years.

Sadly for most of them (until now), if their underlying thyroid condition isn't discovered early in life, they wind up being classified by their doctors as hypochondriacs and written off.

These low-thyroid/low-energy individuals are the best candidates for being overweight. It seems that every mouthful they eat turns to fat or causes fluid retention. They ask themselves, "Why is it so much easier to put on weight than to lose it?"

They turn to ever more restrictive diets and weight-loss panaceas. They shuffle from one type of diet to another—from high-complex carbohydrate to high-protein/low-carbohydrate, to high-fat/low-protein.

And all the diets work—up to a point: the setpoint or plateau (to be covered later). Unfortunately, the best slenderizing efforts of hypothyroids prove to be none too good. Slowly, they drift from doing something to doing nothing.

They begin to view each weight-loss plan as just another

scam. What they don't understand is that losing weight and not gaining it again in all the old familiar places is more than a matter of taking in fewer calories than are expended.

MAKE YOUR THYROID GLAND PERFORM

If you are hypothyroid, how can you assure that your thyroid gland will function normally so that you can lose excessive weight?

In two ways: by specific changes or additions to your diet, or by taking natural, desiccated thyroid prescribed by your doctor.

Dr. Barnes made available to me statistics from patients' case records for an entire generation. They show that first-generation hypothyroids usually can correct their condition simply by adding more iodine-containing foods to their diet: seafood (particularly shrimp)—lobster and crab, as well as saltwater fish (haddock, cod, herring, and halibut). The best food supplements for iodine content are kelp and cod liver oil. (Don't automatically say "yuck" at cod liver oil and refuse to take it. This food supplement now comes in such cover-up flavors as mint, cherry, and strawberry.)

I am often asked on TV and radio talk shows why 40 percent of the population is hypothyroid when table salt is liberally laced with iodine—10 mcg per 100 grams.

Most of us take in enough iodine in salt to prevent goiter, just one sign of thyroid disease. Lack of a goiter doesn't mean that you're home free, as doctors with a depth of experience in this ailment soon learned. However, it would not be sensible to ingest enough salt to prevent hypothyroidism, since too much salt upsets the sodium/potassium balance and can contribute to such serious disorders as edema, insomnia, heart disease, high blood pressure, and obesity.

SAFEST SOURCE OF IODINE

The Recommended Dietary Allowance (RDA) for iodine is 100 micrograms for women and 120 mcg for men. It is unwise and could be hazardous to your health to take in more than this amount in organic form. Kelp tablets are your best and safest supplementary source of iodine.

However, there could be much more to assuring normal thyroid function than merely adding iodine to your diet. Several of my patients learned this the hard way by trying to lose unwanted weight on a strict vegetarian diet accenting soybeans, cabbage, spinach, turnips, and rutabagas, all of which block iodine absorption and, consequently, diminish production of thyroid hormones.

Furthermore, when vegetarians are not secreting sufficient thyroid hormones, the vitamin A precursor in vegetables (carotene) cannot readily be translated into usable vitamin A.

CARE AND FEEDING OF THE THYROID

An entire chapter of our previous book, *Solved: The Riddle of Illness*, was devoted to the care and feeding of thyroid. Here are the major factors to consider.

Two weeks of vitamin A deficiency reduced thyroid hormone secretion of animals by 40 to 50 percent, it was found by Danish biochemist Palludan. (Five thousand I.U. is the recommended daily allowance set by the National Research Council. Illness, trauma, pregnancy, and lactation increase the requirements.)

Likewise, a deficiency in vitamin B-2 depresses the thyroid gland's function, reducing the amount of hormones secreted. Excellent sources of this vitamin are: beef liver, beef heart, almonds, dry nonfat milk and—richest of all—brewer's yeast. Make sure your thyroid gland is fed sufficient vitamin B-6, plentiful in beef liver, kidney, leg of veal, fresh fish, bananas, avocado, walnuts, raisins, prunes, and, especially, wheat germ. Otherwise, it will be handicapped in efforts to convert iodine into thyroid hormones.

Keep your thyroid well fed, along with the rest of you. If you don't, you will have trouble utilizing one of the most hard-to-absorb vitamins: B-12. And enter strict vegetarianism with caution! Such a diet does not contain enough vitamin B-12, obtainable mainly from animal products.

Vitamin B-12 is essential to forming nucleic acid, DNA and RNA, metabolizing carbohydrates, fat, and protein, and keeping nerve tissue healthy. It also helps iron make its contribution to life and health, and assists folic acid (derived from vegetables) to synthesize choline.

Deprive your body of sufficient vitamin C—the RDA of 60 mg seems inadequate to many nutrition authorities—and you could cause bleeding of the thyroid gland, writes Isobel Jennings in *Vitamins in Endocrine Metabolism*, a classic book.[5] Longstanding vitamin C deficiency caused abnormal cell multiplication in guinea pigs, writes Jennings. (Authorities differ as to the appropriate daily amount. Some advocate anywhere from 1,000 mg daily to 18,000 mg. My patients seem to thrive on 1,000 to 4,000 mg daily.)

When rabbits were given subnormal amounts of vitamin E, normal thyroid gland cells multiplied at an abnormal rate and the pituitary, the quarterback of the glandular team, failed to synthesize sufficient thyroid-stimulating hormone (TSH). The result is too little thyroid hormone released, and consequent hypothyroidism. (The RDA for adults is 12 to 15 I.U. daily. Again, many authorities recommend at least 200 I.U. daily.)

Insufficient vitamins are not the only reasons for an underactive thyroid gland. Various drugs and chemicals suppress the thyroid—among them, sulfa drugs and antidiabetic agents. Prednisone and estrogen in pharmacologic doses worsen already unbalanced thyroid function. Thyocyanide in cigarette smoke and fluoride in drinking water inhibit working of the thyroid gland.

BEST BET FOR SECOND GENERATION HYPOTHYROIDS

Second generation hypothyroids usually cannot supplement their thyroid glands successfully with iodine and other nutrients, according to Dr. Barnes. Raw glandular thyroid sold in nutrition centers works for them in some instances. However, their best bet is natural, desiccated thyroid, prescribed by a doctor. Any preventive-medicine specialist or nutrition-oriented medical doctor knows of the Barnes Basal Temperature Test and can prescribe thyroid properly.

Since thyroid hormone is a powerful agent, I start all patients who require it on the equivalent of ¼ to ½ grain of Armour desiccated thyroid preparation daily, increasing the dosage by ¼ to ½ grain every seven to ten days until I achieve desired clinical results. (If Armour is not available, have your doctor prescribe another brand-name, natural preparation.)

I have all my patients check their basal temperature before each office visit. I do not increase their dosage if their basal temperature rises above 98.2 or if their resting heartbeat goes above 85 per minute, or if they experience jitteriness or palpitations. Such symptoms are rarely encountered, however.

Since most of my patients do well on one or two grains, I rarely have to go higher. The limit in my practice has been four grains. When my patients show symptomatic improvement on a proper thyroid dosage, I keep them there and check them every two or three months.

UNDERCOVER MENACE

We have written at length about how the thyroid gland is one of the body's master glands and how hypothyroidism is a common, unsuspected cause of major illness and, occasionally, obesity.

Another common affliction involving the thyroid is Hashimoto's Disease or Autoimmune Thyroiditis (HAIT). It seems incredible that a condition so little known occurs in at least 2 percent of the population, according to an article in *Medical Clinics of North America*. Of the 2 percent, 95 percent are women, making this disease seem discriminatory against women.[6]

My experience and that of other physicians, as well as endocrinologists with whom I have compared notes, is that the

2 percent figure is greatly underestimated. This is unfortunate, because HAIT can block serious weight-loss campaigns.

In different stages of this serious illness, a person can manifest symptoms of either hypothyroidism or hyperthyroidism. Several pages ago, we listed symptoms of hypothyroidism. The classic symptoms of thyroiditis in descending order of frequency are: (1) profound fatigue, (2) memory loss, (3) depression, (4) nervousness, (5) allergies, (6) heartbeat irregularity, (7) muscle and joint pain, (8) sleep disturbances, (9) reduced sex drive, (10) menstrual problems, (11) suicidal tendencies, (12) digestive disorders, (13) headaches and ear pain, (14) lump in the throat, and (15) problems swallowing.

Nervousness ranges from mild anxiety to full-blown panic attacks, of which some are true psychiatric emergencies. These are as puzzling to the patients as to their physicians, who, in desperation, recommend psychotherapy and powerful tranquilizers.

As with anxiety and panic attacks, patients tell me, "I feel so depressed, but I have no reason to feel that way. I have a loving husband, a good job, and caring friends. Something's wrong physically. I know that. Yet all my exams seem normal."

Several of my new patients have admitted becoming so desperate that they had voluntarily signed into psychiatric hospitals for fear of harming themselves. As in anxiety, the treatment of choice in patients with chronic depression in whom thyroiditis goes undiagnosed is powerful antidepressants—which, quite often, make their thyroiditis worse.

Since deep fatigue and psychological problems are the most prevalent complaints of patients with HAIT, their condition, most of the time, is hypothyroidism.

What do you think they do to make themselves feel better?

Right! They eat, gain weight, and can't lose, which adds to their physiologic depression. There are good reasons why I'm writing about HAIT in such detail. The routine blood tests done by your family physician will often show you within normal limits. The Barnes Basal Temperature Test may indicate hypo-

range.

If you suspect that HAIT is your problem, don't fail to corroborate a presumptive diagnosis of this ailment with the following: (1) special immunologic thyroid tests (specifically, the antimicrosomal antibody test), (2) the anti-thyroglobulin antibody test, (3) the thyroid-stimulating immunoglobulin test (TSI), or the thyrotropin-binding Inhibitory Immunoglobulin Test (TBII).

Thyroiditis is a disease of contradictions. Usually any elevation of antithyroid antibodies is significant, if you also have some of the above symptoms. However, in severe cases, you may even have low antithyroid antibodies and, in a mild case, elevated antibodies.

Therefore, I will treat patients medically for thyroiditis with *any* elevation of antithyroid antibodies, if they are also symptomatic. I emphasize this point because many physicians only will treat a case of thyroiditis if they consider the blood antibody level significantly elevated.

In rare instances, patients have all the symptoms of thyroiditis but show normal blood antithyroid antibodies. Fortunately, there are other ways to pinpoint this ailment, through tests for an elevated thyroid-stimulating immunoglobulin (TSI), or a thyrotropin-binding inhibitory immunoglobulin (TBII), or both, or a low basal temperature.

Should you and your physician decide to pursue the diagnosis of HAIT, be sure to have him order all tests from an immunologic testing laboratory. Nichols Institute specializes in this area: Phone: 1 (800) 432-3547 (California) or 1 (800) 854-7197 (all other states).

In addition, have him order a T4, T3, FT1 and T3RIA and a sensitive TSH (also from Nichols). Most of my patients *who are actively being treated* for thyroiditis have been able to resume normal lives and control their weight merely by restricting calories and getting plenty of exercise.

Although my treatment for hypothyroidism is Armour Desiccated Thyroid, I always begin treating thyroiditis patients with

Synthroid, starting with 0.025 mg., which is the equivalent of ¼ grain of desiccated thyroid.

Therapy for thyroiditis doesn't always proceed smoothly. More often it's a case of two steps forward and one step back, with symptoms waxing and waning but usually abating over time. This is why doctors should monitor the condition closely and persist in the proper treatment.

Because of their illness, thyroiditis patients tend to have a weakened immune system. Therefore, it is imperative that they be treated coincidentally for any infections such as chronic Candidiasis—a common problem to be covered in detail in the next chapter—and for food and environmental allergies.

I have gone on at great length about thyroiditis because it is so widespread and often undiagnosed and, most important, because many of my thyroiditis patients *cannot lose weight until thyroiditis is treated successfully*.

An overwhelming majority of my overweight patients are either suffering from hypothyroidism and/or thyroiditis. And they have trouble losing weight until properly diagnosed and treated.

Donna Maria, forty-seven, is an example of hundreds of women I have treated for HAIT over the years. She came to me complaining of a two-year history of severe depression alternating with anxiety attacks. During this time she had been hospitalized for six months in a psychiatric unit and treated with lithium, a major antidepressant, and thirteen episodes of shock therapy.

The latter caused a severe memory loss. In the year before I saw her, she had ballooned fifty pounds with no change in her food intake.

She had low basal temperature, but tests mentioned earlier revealed abnormal thyroid antibodies, for which I started her on Synthroid.

Along with this medication, I upgraded her diet—more protein, vitamins, and minerals—and discontinued her antidepressants. Within ninety days all of her psychiatric symptoms began improving. She lost ten pounds the first month and seven the second; she continues to lose slowly and steadily to this day.

Donna Maria's case is characteristic of untold numbers of women and men who are needlessly, chronically ill and overweight because of an undiagnosed thyroid disorder.

Make sure your thyroid function is normal or compensate for subnormality or abnormality, preferably with your nutrition-oriented, medical doctor's help. Otherwise, your Battle of the Bulge could end up as the 100 Years War. This is the first step in Dr. Langer's weight-loss program.

Others will follow. The second step is discovering whether or not you have Candida albicans and, if so, how it originates, what it does to you weightwise and otherwise, and how to correct it once and for all.

3 | The Yeast Crisis and Overweight

Ailments experienced over several years by plump, thirty-two-year-old Nedra seemed to span the alphabet of medical disorders, from allergies to zeismus.

"I'm desperate," she told me. "Every doctor treats my worst symptom, and if that goes away, something just as bad or worse replaces it. I'm sick and tired of being sick and tired. I want to be healthy and to lose twenty-five pounds."

Nedra had had a series of respiratory infections, for which previous doctors had prescribed antibiotics. Her most recent complaints—anal and vaginal infection, deep fatigue, intermittent depression and overweight—were different faces of the same disorder: Candida albicans, a stubborn fungus that thrives in such warm, moist places as the anus, intestines, nose, throat, and vagina.

Some fifty-five symptoms of this ailment are named by William G. Crook, M.D., in his best-selling book, *The Yeast Connection*.

I dealt with Nedra's condition by the process of elimination: removing junk foods from her diet, particularly those loaded with sugar, which like other refined carbohydrates offers a feast for this fungus and encourages its rapid overgrowth.

Aside from the obvious sugar-laden foods to be avoided— sweet rolls, cake, pies, candy, and ice cream—are the not so obvious ones: processed, packaged, and canned foods, most of which have more hidden sugars than you would imagine.

I pointed out to Nedra that antibiotics had done a number

on her while clearing up her respiratory infections. They had annihilated her gastrointestinal tract's friendly bacteria, which usually dominate and monitor the growth of the yeast. Then, with lactobacillus acidophilus capsules, she eventually recolonized her intestines with friendly microorganisms.

Several months later, the anal and vaginal infections, deep fatigue, and depression left her. Most exciting to her was losing 26 pounds with no conscious effort on her part to diet.

RESISTS DIAGNOSIS

Trying to diagnose Candida albicans by a single culture is a futile exercise because almost everyone is a host for this ubiquitous yeast. I usually follow the game plan of clinical ecologists, which involves taking cultures from a variety of body areas: the anus, armpits, under the breasts, groin, gums, mouth, male genitals, nose, rectum, skin lesions, vagina, and vulva. Wide distribution of the yeast and a heavy overgrowth are key signs of candidiasis.

Another means of confirming the presence of this yeast is a blood test for candida precipitins or antibodies. If the yeast antibodies are elevated and the test is positive, the yeast infection is active and threatening. Conversely, after successful treatment, candida precipitins usually return to normal. Laboratory workers should be reminded that fresh cultures may test negative. Therefore, they should be allowed a minimum of three or four days to grow in a special yeast culture medium.

However, the clincher to any diagnosis is not so much what is happening in the laboratory as what is happening in the patient. Therefore, response to trial therapy and vigilantly monitored results are imperative.

CUT OUT THE SWEET STUFF!

The elimination of sugar and other refined carbohydrates, and the use of lactobacillus acidophilus liquid or capsules and plain yogurt, can help stop the Candida albicans army from advancing on many fronts from its initial beachhead in the intestinal tract. Its numbers will shrink as friendly organisms are taken in, and as they multiply to dominate once more.

Is Candida albicans a new disease?

No. It has been with us since there were yeasts and people on earth. However, Candida albicans was a rare disorder until a generation ago, when special conditions made it possible for these normally quiescent forms of life to become dominant in some individuals:

1. Introduction and increased use of antibiotics since World War II;

2. Utilization of high doses of cortisone;

3. Vastly increased consumption of refined carbohydrates, particularly refined sugar (an estimated 120 pounds per capita each year) and

4. Widespread use of the birth-control pill.

YEAST PIONEERS

C. Orian Truss, M.D., of Birmingham, Alabama, first alerted the world to this now common (but not always recognized) ailment whose time had come. In a series of articles in the *Journal of Orthomolecular Psychiatry* from 1978 through 1984 and also in his enlightening book, *The Missing Diagnosis* (Birmingham, Alabama, 1983), Dr. Truss revealed the relationship of Candida albicans to myriad chronic illnesses that defied diagnosis.

Additionally, pioneering work by Sidney M. Baker, M.D., of New Haven, Connecticut, followed by clinical discoveries by William G. Crook, M.D., related in his runaway best-seller, *The Yeast Connection*, helped make the world aware that dozens of symptoms whose origins were foggy are attributable to Candida albicans.

These doctors, who deserve a special salute from mankind, point out that yeasts are everywhere: airborne, and brought into the body by breathing, and on or in a multitude of ingested foods.

No one is isolated from their invasion, from the newborn babe after its first outcry to the doddering centenarian only a few breaths away from the grave.

Candida albicans is a serious illness. It can make your life miserable, help to add and retain unwelcome weight, and, in extreme cases, even kill.

TAKE A BOW, DR. CROOK!

I am most grateful to Dr. Crook for having alerted me to the widespread prevalence of Candida albicans while a guest on my *Medicine Man* TV program.

Once alerted to this yeast-related ailment, I was able to treat it successfully in scores of patients. In my case experiences, Candida albicans is more common in women than in men, perhaps by a margin of two and one-half to one. The one physical symptom characteristic of young to post-menopausal women is overweight—anywhere from 15 to 50 pounds.

A thirty-four-year-old female patient, after having lost twenty-nine pounds—weight that had stayed off for a year at this writing—remarked with a laugh:

"Losing weight was easy once I followed your Treatment Plan."

Any success I have had in treating Candida albicans—my batting average is 1,000—belongs to William G. Crook, M.D.

THE LESSER CAUSES

It could be that your excess fat padding may be due to the major causes of candida albicans—antibiotics (particularly tetracycline) that can't always be avoided, cortisone, the Pill, overuse of refined carbohydrates, or a bit of each. Or it could be from less well-known causes:

1. Diabetes mellitus (high blood sugar level).
2. Pregnancy (one or more).
3. Malnutrition.

4. Overeating.
5. Chemotherapy.
6. Debilitating illness.
7. Radiation.

Why do these factors encourage the overgrowth of the Candida albicans yeast? No one knows for sure. However, it seems that they contribute their own particular form of stress.

Now that you know something about Candida albicans, you may be wondering if there's a simple way to determine whether or not this is your problem. Unfortunately, overweight—the beginning indicator—is ambiguous, since excess poundage can result from any number of causes.

ARE *YOU* A CANDIDA CANDIDATE?

So let's start on a more firm foundation. Let's review *Dr. Crook's Candida Questionnaire and Score Sheet*, which he permitted us to utilize.

CANDIDA QUESTIONNAIRE
AND SCORE SHEET

This questionnaire is designed for adults and the scoring system isn't appropriate for children. It lists factors in your medical history which promote the growth of Candida albicans (Section A), and symptoms commonly found in individuals with yeast-connected illness (Section B and C).

For each "Yes" answer in Section A, circle the Point Score in that section. Total your score and record it in the box at the end of the section. Then move on to Sections B and C and score as directed.

Filling out and scoring this questionnaire should help you and your physician evaluate the possible role of Candida in contributing to your health problems. Yet it will not provide an automatic "Yes" or "No" answer.

The Candida questionnaire and score sheet is reproduced in full from THE YEAST CONNECTION by William G. Crook, M.D., Future Health, Inc., 681 Skyline Drive, Jackson, Tennessee 38301. Used with permission.

This questionnaire is available in quantity from Professional Books, P.O. Box 3494, Jackson, Tennessee 38301. Prices on request.
Copyright ©, 1983, William G. Crook, M.D.

SECTION A: HISTORY

Point/Score

---

1. Have you taken tetracyclines (Sumycin®, Pan-mycin®, Vibramycin®, Minocin®, etc.) or other antibiotics for acne for 1 month (or longer)? **35**

---

2. Have you, at any time in your life, taken other "broad spectrum" antibiotics† for respiratory, urinary or other infections (for 2 months or longer, or in shorter courses 4 or more times in a 1-year period?) **35**

---

3. Have you taken a broad spectrum antibiotic drug†—even a single course? **6**

---

4. Have you, at any time in your life, been bothered by persistent prostatitis, vaginitis or other problems affecting your reproductive organs? **25**

---

5. Have you been pregnant . . .
2 or more times? **5**

1 time? **3**

---

6. Have you taken birth control pills . . .
For more than 2 years? **15**

For 6 months to 2 years? **8**

---

7. Have you taken prednisone, Decadron® or other cortisone-type drugs . . .
For more than 2 weeks? **15**

For 2 weeks or less? **6**

---

† Including Keflex,® ampicillin, amoxicillin, Ceclor,® Bactrim® and Septra®. Such antibiotics kill off "good germs" while they're killing off those which cause infection.

8. Does exposure to perfumes, insecticides, fabric shop odors and other chemicals provoke . . .

Moderate to severe symptoms?	20
Mild symptoms?	5

9. Are your symptoms worse on damp, muggy days or in moldy places? | 20

10. Have you had athlete's foot, ring worm, "jock itch" or other chronic fungous infections of the skin or nails? Have such infections been . . .

Severe or persistent?	20
Mild to moderate?	10

11. Do you crave sugar?	10
12. Do you crave breads?	10
13. Do you *crave alcoholic beverages?*	10
14. Does tobacco smoke *really* bother you?	10

Total Score, Section A . . . .————

SECTION B: MAJOR SYMPTOMS:

For each of your symptoms, enter the appropriate figure in the Point Score column:

If a symptom is *occasional or mild* . . . score 3 points
If a symptom is *frequent and/or moderately severe* . . .
score 6 points
If a symptom is *severe and/or disabling* . score 9 points
Add total score and record it in the box at the end of this section.
Point/Score

1. Fatigue or lethargy

2. Feeling of being "drained"

3. Poor memory

4. Feeling "spacey" or "unreal"

5. Inability to make decisions

6. Numbness, burning or tingling

7. Insomnia

8. Muscle aches

9. Muscle weakness or paralysis

10. Pain and/or swelling in joints

11. Abdominal pain

12. Constipation

13. Diarrhea

14. Bloating, belching or intestinal gas

15. Troublesome vaginal burning, itching or discharge

16. Prostatitis

17. Impotence

18. Loss of sexual desire or feeling

19. Endometriosis or infertility

20. Cramps and/or other menstrual irregularities

21. Premenstrual tension

22. Attacks of anxiety or crying

23. Cold hands or feet and/or chilliness

24. Shaking or irritable when hungry

Total Score, Section B . . . .——

SECTION C: OTHER SYMPTOMS:†

For each of your symptoms, enter the appropriate figure in the Point Score column:

      If a symptom is *occasional or mild* . . . score 1 points

      If a symptom is *frequent and/or moderately severe* . . .

                                      score 2 points

      If a symptom is *severe and/or disabling* . score 3 points

Add total score and record it in the box at the end of this section.

                                          Point/Score

1. Drowsiness
2. Irritability or jitteriness
3. Incoordination
4. Inability to concentrate
5. Frequent mood swings
6. Headache
7. Dizziness/loss of balance
8. Pressure above ears . . . feeling of head swelling
9. Tendency to bruise easily
10. Chronic rashes or itching
11. Numbness, tingling
12. Indigestion or heartburn
13. Food sensitivity or intolerance
14. Mucus in stools
15. Rectal itching
16. Dry mouth or throat
17. Rash or blisters in mouth
18. Bad breath

†While the symptoms in this section commonly occur in people with yeast-connected illness they are also found in other individuals.

19. Foot, hair or body odor not relieved by washing

20. Nasal congestion or post nasal drip

21. Nasal itching

22. Sore throat

23. Laryngitis, loss of voice

24. Cough or recurrent bronchitis

25. Pain or tightness in chest

26. Wheezing or shortness of breath

27. Urinary frequency or urgency

28. Burning on urination

29. Spots in front of eyes or erratic vision

30. Burning or tearing of eyes

31. Recurrent infections or fluid in ears

32. Ear pain or deafness

Total Score, Section C . . . .———

Total Score, Section A . . . .———

Total Score, Section B . . . .———

GRAND TOTAL SCORE . . . .———

The Grand Total Score will help you and your physician decide if your health problems are yeast-connected. Scores in women will run higher as 7 items in the questionnaire apply exclusively to women, while only 2 apply exclusively to men.

Yeast-connected health problems are almost certainly present in women with scores *over 180*, and in men with scores *over 140*.

Yeast-connected health problems are probably present in women with scores *over 120* and in men with scores *over 90*.

Yeast-connected health problems are possibly present in women with scores *over 60* and in men with scores *over 40*.

With scores of less than 60 in women and 40 in men, yeasts are less apt to cause health problems.

If your questionnaire score came up on the Candida albicans side, there are several corrective measures you can take—preferably under guidance of a medical doctor who understands Candida albicans, a clinical ecologist, or a nutritionally oriented physician.

No therapy will guarantee your being well overnight; it could take many months. Before listing my specific regime, let me mention that in extreme cases, I prescribe Nystatin, an effective, anti-fungal medication derived from a soil mold. This annihilates yeasts on contact. Its other advantages are that little is absorbed into the bloodstream, and it is safe for most persons. (I have had only two patients who could not tolerate it.)

CONQUERING CANDIDA

However, my favored treatment is nonmedical, accenting nutrition. This calls for a radical change in life-style. I recommend that you:

1. Stop eating sugar—white, brown, corn syrup, honey, maple syrup, or molasses—and sugared products, as well as milk, cheese, fruit, and bakery goods (especially those made from refined flour). My Mega-Weight Loss Diet in the last chapter includes whole-grain breads and muffins in moderate amounts. However, these can be baked without yeast. (Milk and yeast-containing foods do not always cause or encourage overgrowth of Candida, but they often cause food sensitivities and allergies, which can produce symptoms similar to those of Candida. They should be omitted from the diet for at least three weeks and then added singly and monitored to see if they produced marked physiological reactions before being reinstated.)

2. Eat plentiful vegetables, whole grains, meat (chicken and lamb), fish, nuts, butter, cold-pressed oils, and sugarless, fruitless yogurt—the latter to reinforce your defending army of friendly bacteria. (Many milk-intolerants can tolerate yogurt.)

3. Add food supplements to your daily diet, my anti-Candida albicans regime:

Two tablespoons of liquid lactobacillus acidophilus before each meal. (This is one of the major types of friendly bacteria that helps keep Candida albicans yeast in check.)

Six squirts of liquid, odorless garlic from the squeezable, plastic bottle in a half glass of water, twice daily.

Two 500 mg gamma-linolenic acid (GLA) tablets three times daily.

A good multiple vitamin that contains minerals.

A vitamin B-complex pill (50 mg of the major B fractions) to compensate for reduced capacity of the declining colony of friendly intestinal bacteria to synthesize certain members of this vitamin family.

4 grams (a level teaspoon) of granular vitamin C daily. (I start children and teenagers on ⅛ teaspoon, gradually going up to ¼ teaspoon, then ½. Anyone who takes this should stop at the level before diarrhea occurs.)

Two cups of Pau D'Arco tea daily. Commonly called Taheebo tea, this product can be bought at most nutrition centers.

4. Abstain from all forms of alcohol. Refrain from smoking and abuse of drugs. (4a) Capristatin (gen Caprilic acid) or 1 Tab 3 × /D (available a.t.c. at nutrition centers).

5. Tune up your body and strengthen your immune system with regular exercise.

6. Work closely with your doctor and enlist the cooperation of your mate or other family members in menu planning.

DIETARY DOs AND DON'Ts

Eating fruits promotes yeast growth because fruits are loaded with fructose, which is readily converted to simple sugars in the intestinal tract.

Dr. Crook rules out all fruit juices in his therapy—canned, bottled, frozen—because of their high sugar content and because some of the fruit used in juicing is overripe and may contain mold.

So do I.

All processed foods are omitted during therapy—bottled, boxed, canned, and packaged—and, I hope, from this point on.

Cheese, especially the moldy ones like Roquefort and bleu, is verboten, as are cheese-laden snacks. Peanuts, too, are forbidden, because often they are contaminated with aspergillus mold—again, not because one form of yeast or mold encourages another such as Candida albicans, but because many persons are sensitive or allergic to them.

With so many dietary "don'ts," how can a person find some "dos"?

Not easily. However, conquering Candida albicans is worth the effort, as a number of my patients have told me. Until the Candida albicans is under control, it is best to eat proteins, complex carbohydrate foods and low-carbohydrate-content vegetables, seeds, and nuts.

Later, it will be possible to add small portions of the lowest carbohydrate-content fruits.

This seemingly severe regime works. It conquers Candida albicans and its host of unpleasant symptoms.

Best of all, it helps to dissolve unwanted fat and make clothing fit like garments, rather than strait jackets.

And, after all, isn't that the name of the game?

4 | Killing Me Sweetly

Like Candida albicans, reactive hypoglycemia (low blood sugar) could be one of the subtle saboteurs of your weight-loss program. On the surface, this may seem strange because hypoglycemia is far more notorious for sapping victims with weakness, exhaustion, and faintness.

However, don't make the mistake of ruling it out until you check it out—preferably with a nutritionally oriented doctor. I make this recommendation because most physicians still don't believe there is such a disorder.

I do after having treated more than 100 cases with diet. And I also have observed in my patients that hypoglycemia contributes to overweight and even to obesity.

Some years ago, after patients had lost considerable weight with the correction of their low blood sugar, I thought I had made a significant discovery.

Then someone shattered my illusion by showing me an article, "Low Blood Sugar Can Make You Fat" in the *Encylopedia of Common Diseases* by the staff of *Prevention Magazine*, published by Rodale Press. The gist of it was this: loading the bloodstream with refined carbohydrates causes reactive hypoglycemia, a condition in which blood sugar drops sharply, and the person has candy or a cup of coffee to recharge him or herself. The article stated that this kind of individual is tired, miserable, hungry all the time, and prone to weight gain.

HOW HYPOGLYCEMIA WORKS

To understand better how this enemy within works, let's first review what hypoglycemia is. Although authorities have differences—so what else is new?—many of them maintain that this disorder results from the manner in which the body handles or mishandles sugar, instead of just the amount of sugar in the bloodstream at any particular time.

When a non-hypoglycemic person eats a sugar-laden candy bar, the glucose (sugar) in his or her blood rises until insulin, a hormone secreted by the pancreas, is slowly released, reducing the glucose—an energy source—to the fasting level, the point at which hunger demands attention.

Things are just the opposite when a hungry hypoglycemic wolfs a candy bar. His or her pancreas suffers shock and over-reacts, releasing so much insulin into the blood that sugar is removed too quickly, creating a deficit of glucose and initiating new hunger. This is a demonstration of reactive hypoglycemia.

Repeated assaults with refined sugar (in candy, cookies, cake, rolls, and ice cream, or stirred into coffee or tea) or starches make the pancreas trigger-happy, increasing hunger and causing hypoglycemics to eat often—usually the wrong foods, simple carbohydrates, which give them more calories than they need for sustenance.

These calories are converted to fat and go to waist, hips, and/or thighs. Right after a gooey piece of cake, full of refined sugar and flour that are quickly absorbed, your blood sugar leaps high, and you feel all's right with the world. Then comes the big insulin surge, your blood sugar drops, and you plunge from the mountain top to the pits.

All the cells of your body and brain cry out for more fuel; you begin to drag, feel light-headed, irritable, nervous, and/or depressed. These and other negative, "downer" symptoms make you want to eat to be good to yourself.

So that you understand hypoglycemia better and can find out whether or not it is keeping you overweight, let's consider more in depth what happens when you eat and digest food and it ends up as glucose.

Your body's "traffic coordinator" routes the glucose through the bloodstream directly to the liver. If it weren't for the liver, the sugar from one meal would send your blood sugar so high that you would be a diabetic.

This is where the hormone insulin comes in. As the glucose-carrying blood exits from the liver into the bloodstream, the upward charge of blood sugar activates the pancreas to release insulin into the circulating blood, where, after making the rounds, the glucose enters the liver. The liver then does one of its major jobs: transforming glucose into storable glycogen.

Preventing too much glucose from circulating, the insulin performs still another critical function: it helps each fuel-hungry cell to receive and burn the glucose for heat and energy.

Although the body can endure excessive sugar levels for a time, it is stressed by insufficient sugar levels. However, either of these conditions indicates an imbalance of the energy use system.

LITTLE-CONSIDERED CAUSES

To attribute all hypoglycemia to hypersensitivity to carbohydrate shock would be an oversimplification. Several other conditions can depress sugar levels: some drugs; deficiency of the B-complex family of vitamins (particularly B-1 and B-2 and niacin, essential to efficient carbohydrate metabolism); a deficiency of protein (this, along with a shortage of pantothenic acid and vitamin B-2 can frustrate the liver's efforts to inactivate excess insulin); sustained stress; tired adrenal glands; a pancreatic tumor (which stimulates insulin production); food allergies; and hypothyroidism.

Constant stress overworks the adrenal glands to prepare us for "fight or flight" by triggering their secretion of adrenalin, which sets off a glandular sequence that translates glycogen stores in the liver into blood sugar.

Alcohol, coffee, caffeine-containing colas, and smoking or chewing tobacco all stimulate the adrenals to the same stresslike action.

Hypothyroidism also tilts the delicate balance of the adrenal glands. Insufficient thyroid hormone in the bloodstream causes the adrenal glands to slow down their secretion of cortisol (hydrocortisone). Since cortisol stimulates the liver's production of glycogen, hypothyroidism can indirectly—but just as seriously—cause hypoglycemia.

The Thyroid, a prestigious text edited by Sidney Werner, M.D., and Sidney H. Ingbar, M.D., cites an animal experiment in which hypothyroidism caused the adrenal glands to waste away. Research in relation to human beings is not quite so conclusive.

YOUR LIVER: AN INCREDIBLE PERFORMER

Along with the thyroid and adrenal glands, the liver must work properly to keep carbohydrate metabolism in balance. In hypothyroids, the liver is sluggish and stores glucose too slowly. Then blood sugar may be deceptively high in a fasting glucose tolerance test. Additionally, under these circumstances, an individual may get rid of this excess glucose in the urine and unjustifiably be labeled a prediabetic.

Old Man Liver, he just keeps rollin' along, if properly nourished. If not, he develops all sorts of problems: accumulation of fat, scar tissue, cirrhosis, and reduction of enzymes and coenzymes so that foods cannot be properly metabolized.

The body's second largest organ (largest is the skin), located right above the stomach, the liver is a virtual industrial plant where chemical reactions by the thousands happen with lightning rapidity.

The liver's job description is amazing. This one organ:

- Produces amino acids (building blocks of protein), utilizing them to make living tissue;

- Breaks down protein into sugar for energy, and into fat in overeating;

- Synthesizes prothrombin, which makes possible the clotting of blood;

- Helps produce bile, blood albumin, cholesterol, and lecithin;

- Transforms dietary sugar into glycogen, which it stores, changing it back to blood sugar as required;

- Stores copper, iron, various trace minerals, vitamin A, and, to a lesser degree, vitamins D, E, and K as well as (only briefly) some B vitamins;

- Inactivates excess hormones, destroys histamines, rids us of certain harmful metals, chemicals, and drugs, and detoxifies us of poisons and toxins.

The liver must function efficiently to help prevent hypoglycemia and weight gain or weight retention by its ability to form and store glycogen and provide needed energy and stamina. If it produces too little insulinase, the pancreas secretes too much insulin.

Fortunately, even much-abused livers can make a remarkable comeback on a diet right in complete protein and in B-complex vitamins, as well as vitamin C, choline, and vitamin E.

An experiment was conducted with 102 individuals whose diet had been habitually high in refined carbohydrates and very low in protein, resulting in development of enlarged, fatty, and painful livers.

Their diet was enhanced with more protein, and with supplements of choline, methionine, and vitamin B-12. Weekly needle biopsies noted improvements in the liver. Every patient recovered within six weeks.

It is apparent then: as goes your liver, so goes your carbohydrate metabolism and your chance of defeating hypoglycemia and, of major importance, losing burdensome weight.

CHECK YOURSELF FOR LOW BLOOD SUGAR

Probably the most comprehensive survey of hypoglycemia symptoms was done by Stephen Gyland, M.D., of Jacksonville, Florida. His review of 600 well-documented hypoglycemics revealed the following most common symptoms and the percentages of persons with each complaint.

See how you rate:

Nervousness	94 percent.
Irritability	89 percent.
Exhaustion	87 percent.
Faintness, dizziness, tremor, cold sweats, weak spells	86 percent.
Depression	77 percent.
Vertigo, dizziness	73 percent.
Drowsiness	72 percent.
Headaches	71 percent.
Digestive disturbances	69 percent.
Forgetfulness	67 percent.
Insomnia (awakening and inability to return to sleep)	67 percent.
Constant worrying, unprovoked anxiety	62 percent.
Mental confusion	57 percent.
Palpitation of heart, rapid pulse	54 percent.
Muscle pains	53 percent.
Numbness	51 percent.

| Used with permission of Stephen Gyland, M.D.

Indecisiveness	50 percent.
Unsocial, asocial, and antisocial behavior	47 percent.
Crying spells	46 percent.
Lack of sex drive (females)	44 percent.
Allergies	43 percent.
Lack of coordination	42 percent.
Leg cramps	43 percent.
Blurred vision	40 percent.
Twitching and jerking of muscles	40 percent.
Itching and crawling sensation on skin	39 percent.
Gasping for breath	37 percent.
Smothering spells	34 percent.
Staggering	34 percent.
Sighing and yawning	30 percent.
Impotence (males)	27 percent.
Unconsciousness	27 percent.
Night terrors, nightmares	27 percent.
Rheumatoid arthritis	24 percent.
Phobias, fears	23 percent.
Neurodermatitis	21 percent.

Suicidal intent	20 percent.
Nervous breakdown	17 percent.
Convulsions	2 percent.

MUST WE TOLERATE THE GLUCOSE TOLERANCE TEST?

These symptoms, particularly the first fifteen, can help you determine whether or not you are hypoglycemic. Getting confirmation from your doctor is a good idea. However, his method of arriving at a diagnosis is the five- or six-hour glucose tolerance test, which is not always accurate.

You come to the doctor's office or a laboratory after having fasted overnight, and your fasting blood-sugar level is determined as a base. Then you get a sickeningly sweet dose of sugar (glucose)—about 100 grams (roughly 3½ ounces).

Next your blood sugar is measured, usually twice during the first hour and then every hour until the fifth or sixth hours. Some authorities feel that this test has more liabilities than assets.

If anything, it is unnatural, nothing like conditions in real life. Being fed pure glucose usually has no relation to your regular dietary pattern.

First, the test is usually administered in the quiet of a physician's office or a laboratory. The patient is insulated from his daily exposure to stresses, which influence blood-sugar level. Further, symptoms of hypoglycemia do not always occur conveniently during test measurements. The best time to check blood glucose is when symptoms occur.

Use of glucose can muddy test results, too, since glucose fed to patients is usually derived from corn, one of the top food allergens. Since food sensitivities and allergies are common to hypoglycemics, the question arises: is the patient reacting to glucose or to corn, its food source, or to both?

Add this complicating fact: most hypoglycemics tested are exposed to a combination of glucose and sugar, fructose, sugar from fruits and vegetables, and lactose (milk sugar). Why not test people with sugar, rather than with glucose?

To make the glucose more palatable, some laboratories give it a cola flavor, not considering that many soft drinks contain caffeine, which revs up the adrenal glands to signal the liver to release more sugar into the blood. This is another cause for distorted readings.

Unfortunately, doctors all too often pay more attention to test numbers than to patients' symptoms. I have heard horror stories from a number of patients whose glaring symptoms—bursting into tears, incoherent speech, and even convulsions—were ignored because blood sugar measurements were slightly above the lower limit: 60 milligrams per 100 milliliters of blood.

Such interpretations fail to consider individual variation, as is well demonstrated by the lifelong work of Dr. Roger Williams. I have seen patients go into typical, violent hypoglycemic crying jags when their blood sugar was still above or at the bottom extreme of normal. No matter how sincere the persons who established the line of demarcation between normal and low blood sugar, patients often show the full spectrum of hypoglycemic reactions while just above or at the 60 mg mark. Human metabolism has its own ranges of function, and it does not always suit the convenience of numbers established by researchers.

HOW TO HELP YOUR DOCTOR AND YOURSELF

If you suspect you're hypoglycemic, help your doctor help you. Do some sleuthing. Make a report. Find out at what time of day or night (or both) you usually experience symptoms. Then also write down every food you have eaten on that day and at the approximate time. If you know the specific time when symptoms occur, you can schedule an appointment with your doctor at that time, so that he or she can take your blood sugar reading then.

(At very low cost, you can purchase, with a doctor's prescription, a portable instrument known as a glucometer. With a drop of blood from a fingerstick, you can measure your blood-sugar level day or night. For more information on this and other home tests, the best book on the market is *Do-It-Yourself Medical Testing* (Over 160 Tests You Can Do at Home) by Cathey Pinckney and Edward R. Pinckney, M.D. (Facts on File).

If your symptoms persist despite the doctor's inability to find your blood sugar below the baseline, and the doctor begins to categorize you as a hypochondriac or neurotic, find and consult a nutrition-oriented doctor.

If this fails to work out, you may want to devise your own diet for hypoglycemia—low in simple carbohydrates and high in protein and complex carbohydrates. Here is guidance for your regime:

Foods to Use	Foods to Avoid
Beef, lamb, poultry	Sugar (all forms)
Fish and shellfish	Candies, cake, pastries, pies, dates, raisins
Cheese, milk, yogurt kefir	Macaroni, spaghetti, white rice
All vegetables	
Whole grain cereal and bread	Sweetened soft drinks
Soybeans and their products	Alcohol
Nuts (preferably unsalted)	Coffee
Eggs (unless you are hypercholesterolemic)	Processed cereals
Butter (unless you are hypercholesterolemic)	
Low-carbohydrate fruits	

SIX SMALL MEALS

To keep your blood sugar above the danger area, you may temporarily have to eat five or six small meals daily, using foods in the left column.

My diet permits no canned foods—fruits or vegetables—since most of them contain some form of sugar: corn syrup, cane, or beet.

When you use vegetables and fruit, choose those that are in the low carbohydrate-content groups. Below are carbohydrate values of these foods in descending order:

Dates and figs are so sugar-rich, they should be omitted from the diet of hypoglycemics. In a slightly lower bracket—20 percent—are the major "no-nos": bananas, sweet cherries, grape juice, prunes, and certain beans (kidney, lima and navy), corn, hominy, and sweet potatoes.

In the 15-percent-carbohydrate group—to be eaten sparingly—are apples, apricots, blueberries, sour cherries, currants, grapes, huckleberries, loganberries, nectarines, pears, pineapples, and plums. Vegetables in this group are artichokes, parsnips, and peas.

Among the 10-percent-carbohydrate fruits and vegetables are cantaloupe, oranges, peaches, fresh raspberries, Hubbard squash, and turnips.

I urge my patients to use foods in this group liberally, along with those in the two lowest brackets—7 and 5 percent, respectively. In the 7 percent category are grapefruit, lemons, strawberries, and watermelon, as well as avocados and olives.

Containing 5 percent carbohydrates or less are fresh beans, carrots, cauliflower, okra, onions, pepper, pumpkin, radishes, string beans, and watercress. Sorry, no fruits.

This diet has brought successful control of hypoglycemia to my patients. However, it does even more. It gradually makes them less dependent on refined sugars and starches. In the bargain, it helps melt away unwanted fat.

If this regime doesn't bring relief of your symptoms of hypoglycemia, there's a good chance you are hypothyroid. More than 75 percent of my hypoglycemia patients also are hypothyroid, which is why there's such a tremendous overlap of symptoms.

Of course, you should be treated immediately. A second possibility is that you may be suffering from either food sensitivities or sub-clinical malnutrition. Food sensitivities and allergies are the subject of the next chapter.

5 | Lose Allergies and Weight

Several years ago, my collaborator, health editor/writer James F. Scheer, questioned the findings of clinical ecologists that desisting from allergenic foods often encouraged weight loss.

Then he took a comprehensive food-allergy test, eliminated allergenic foods and, within eight weeks, lost sixteen previously tenacious pounds.

Now this Doubting Thomas is a true believer.

Some of my patients were equally skeptical until they learned two things: (1) that my medical files hold case histories of eighty-four persons who lost from fifteen to fifty pounds by this method, and (2) that this could happen to them.

In the process, they also lost countless hours of sneezing, wheezing, sniffling, stuffy nose, headaches, dry and scratchy throat, generalized itching, and rashes, plus a host of other disagreeable symptoms. Few individuals die from allergies, but millions feel like dying from some of them.

As mentioned in the previous chapter, creating a surefire, anti-hypoglycemia diet is not always possible just by minimizing or eliminating refined carbohydrates and accenting proteins and complex carbohydrates.

PROBLEM FOODS

Such an approach works in many instances. However, it does not account for the fact that permitted foods frequently

include allergens capable of causing hypoglycemia or hyperglycemia (diabetes).

This is not merely my opinion. It is the considered judgment
of psychiatrist William H. Philpott, M.D., who has dedicated
many years to clinical investigation in this field. Much of Dr.
Philpott's study is founded on the solid and abundant research
of several giants among clinical ecologists: Drs. Theron G. Randolph, Max Rinkel, and Marshall Mandell. Some of Philpott's
work was done with Dr. Mandell.

As Dr. Philpott once told me, "A shaky generalization exists
in relation to carbohydrate intolerance. Both the hypoglycemic
(low-blood-sugar person) and the hyperglycemic (diabetic) are
considered to be carbohydrate intolerant, because the five- or six-
hour glucose tolerance test is made with a single carbohydrate
(corn sugar). Blood-sugar levels monitored before and after the
test sample indicate that a patient cannot properly handle sugar.

"Testers generalize from the corn-sugar samples that blood
sugar is too low or too high because of carbohydrate intolerance.
Next comes an often erroneous assumption that, because of the
blood-sugar evidence, all other carbohydrates are not tolerable.
The step beyond this is the faulty conclusion that the proper
treatment of two carbohydrate-intolerant conditions—hypoglycemia and diabetes—should be the minimizing of all carbohydrates.

"Many of us investigators in this area have found the sur-
prising evidence that, in susceptible people, low and high blood
sugar can be evoked by *all* categories of foods and beverages—
fat, proteins, and carbohydrates—as well as chemicals such as
petrochemical hydrocarbons and even tobacco. And, note this
fact particularly: foods lowering or elevating the blood sugar are
specific to each person. Such reactions can be precipitated by
any substance to which a person reacts maladaptively."

(An example of maladaptive reaction among my patients is
the case of Russ, mentioned in Chapter 1.)

"Simply stated, low or high blood-sugar levels can be caused
by specific allergic-like reactions to specific substances," Philpott
added. "The key problem is that hypoglycemia and hypergly-

cemia are not just maladaptive response to a single category of foods (carbohydrates) but to a specific food or chemical that interferes with the complex biochemical mechanisms that are attempting to regulate blood sugar to the proper level.''

Philpott also concluded that exhaust fumes from cars or diesel-powered trucks, or fumes from gas stoves and cleaning solvents, as well as such allergens as pollens, molds, or animal danders, can disturb carbohydrate metabolism and upset the normal balance of blood sugar as well.

You may ask, ''How can specific foods or vapors cause low blood sugar?''

Easily, if you are sensitive or allergic to them. All the answers are not clear yet, but allergens seem to act upon you as stressors, like extreme cold or heat, exhausting exercise, work beyond your physical capacity, personalities abrasive to you, depression, fear, or any ''fight or flight'' situation.

THE PATTERN: HYPOGLYCEMIA TO DIABETES

The stage of stress determines whether a patient suffers from low blood sugar or high blood sugar. According to Dr. Hans Selye, who discovered the famous stress theory, there are three stages in reaction to stressors: (1) alarm (the body is aware of the insult); (2) adaptation (the body tries to adjust to the insult) and (3) exhaustion (the glands involved in the attempted adjustment to continuous or severe stress become over-fatigued or even incapable of further function).

This is a critical issue: hypoglycemia occurs during adaptation to stress of any kind—in this instance, stress to food allergens. Too much insulin is secreted and blood sugar is lowered. Then, as adaptation gives way to exhaustion, the pancreas and related glands and organs involved in sugar metabolism slow down, causing low insulin levels and consequent high blood sugar.

So, according to this theory, the difference between low blood sugar and diabetes is how long the food and/or environmental stressors persist and how resilient are the sugar metabolizing glands and organs. In other words, unless the underlying cause of hypoglycemia is detected and corrected, adult onset diabetes could well follow.

There is no easy answer to what foods or environmental substances you're sensitive to, since most such stressors are subtle. However, pioneering clinical ecologists have made tremendous contributions to understanding sensitivities and allergies to foods and environmental substances, and to developing accurate tests to detect them.

An important early discovery by clinical ecologists was that the scratch or prick-puncture test for food allergies, which is the backbone of traditional allergy medical practice, is only about 20 percent accurate. The late Arthur Coca, M.D., one of the eminent early clinical ecologists, explained that, in order to manifest the typical allergic reaction to food—swelling, redness, or skin elevation like a mosquito bite—the patient had to have blood substances known as reagins, which Dr. Marshall Mandell calls "a kind of allergic antibody which *may be formed* in response to various foods for which a person may be tested."

HOW TO DISCOVER FOOD ALLERGENS

Most individuals don't have reagins.

Some do-it-yourself tests devised by clinical ecologists can help you pinpoint food sensitizing agents: the Coca Pulse Test and the late Dr. Herbert Rinkel's Rotary Diversified Diet.

Dr. Coca, an internationally respected immunologist, honorary president of the American Association of Immunologists and founder and first editor of the *Journal of Immunology*, discovered the important connection between an increased pulse rate and food sensitivities or allergies.

According to Coca, any dramatic rise in heartbeat following food ingestion—20 or more beats higher than normal—is very likely caused by a sensitivity or allergy to food.

How can you take the Coca test?

First, locate the area inside your wrist where you can feel the pulse of blood pumped by your heart. Simply count your pulse for six seconds and multiply by ten to obtain a resting pulse.

Take your pulse reading before getting out of bed in the morning. Do it again just before breakfast. Take your pulse reading thirty minutes after this meal and again sixty minutes after breakfast.

You can test each individual food that you suspect may be bothering you every hour from then on. Your food sensitizing agents or allergens will cause your pulse to speed up, sometimes at a frightening pace. Certain of my patients who use the pulse test have seen their heartbeat rise from 72 to as high as 180 after they have eaten an allergenic food.

Keep an accurate record of the harmful foods and omit them from your diet. I have seen remarkable recoveries from asthma, bronchitis, watery eyes, itchy or inflamed throat, sneezing, wheezing, and coughing when patients have abstained from allergenic foods. However, what seemed to please them most was a dramatic loss in weight.

RINKEL'S REVEALING ROTARY DIVERSIFIED DIET

Before describing Dr. Herbert Rinkel's Rotary Diversified Diet, I should tell you of the several kinds of allergies he discovered: (1) a type dependent on the number of exposures you have to an allergenic food, drink, or chemical substance; (2) addictive allergy; and (3) the "fixed" allergy.

The first kind is self-explanatory. However, addictive allergy could use a bit of comment. This involves eating the same foods frequently, sometimes daily or a number of times daily.

Persons addicted to certain foods are usually not aware of their dependency on them. If they even give the subject a thought, they usually attribute their preference to a natural food craving. It could be more than that. It could be a habituation similar to smoking, coffee drinking, or use of alcohol.

Upon missing a meal that includes the food to which the eater is allergic, he or she experiences withdrawal symptoms. To alleviate the withdrawal reactions, this person will hunger unconsciously for the addictive food. In time, he or she will repeatedly ingest the allergenic food before obvious symptoms appear. This phenomenon was called "masking" by Dr. Rinkel.

The last of the major food-allergy types is the fixed allergy. One has a negative reaction to certain foods whenever they are eaten, even in seemingly trivial amounts. This is the most difficult food allergy problem to deal with.

The Rotary Diversified Diet is based on a revealing discovery by Rinkel. If you avoid allergenic foods for at least four days and then eat them, you suffer from acute and obvious allergic reactions.

To follow this diet, you eat just a single food at a meal and do not eat it again until four days have passed. If sensitive or allergic to it, you will usually experience a marked flare-up of symptoms.

If you are not sensitive to the foods you are testing, your lack of symptoms will tell you to go ahead. Bon appetit! Just repeat the process, trying another food at each meal until you exhaust the list of suspected and unsuspected foods. Soon you will develop a wide range of foods from which you can build your menus.

However, beware of continuous repetition of even harmless foods. If you do, you run the risk of developing new sensitivities or allergies. Rinkel recommends not repeating even the non-allergenic foods any more than every fifth day or more.

The Rotary Diversified Diet offers you two specific benefits. It reveals foods to which you are sensitive or allergic, and then helps keep you from developing new food allergies and addictions.

BEST PLACE TO BEGIN

My advice to patients who would like to uncover their food sensitivities using the Coca Pulse Test and/or the Rinkel Rotary Diversified Diet is, first, to single out foods and beverages they eat most often. These are most likely to be allergenic and addictive.

Another good starting point is the list of foods most commonly found by allergists and clinical ecologists to be allergenic. James Braly, M.D., president of Optimum Health Laboratory in Encino, California, a former student of Dr. Theron Randolph, offers the following suspect foods: corn, yeast, wheat, milk, eggs, soybeans, coffee, citrus fruits, chocolate, tomatoes, potatoes, spices, malt, nuts, beef, and pork.

"Most individuals follow a perfect formula for developing food sensitivities and allergies and reinforcing old ones," according to Dr. Braly. "This is eating only ten to twenty of the same foods day in and day out."

In checking food charts of my allergic and overweight patients, I find that few of them eat more than twenty different foods. This is a practice that I quickly discourage, which usually pays off with the successful disappearance of chronic health complaints and dramatic weight loss.

CAN YOU EVER DE-ALLERGIZE FOOD?

I am frequently asked by patients and radio and TV talk show hosts, "Is it ever possible to reinstate allergenic foods without suffering the consequences of unpleasant symptoms and weight gain?"

Sometimes. After three months of abstinence from allergenic foods, you might want to experiment, adding small amounts of one such food at a time. However, be vigilant for a long laundry list of symptoms: sniffles, sneezes, post-nasal drip, blurred vision, watery eyes, earache, ear infections, headaches (sometimes migraines, as described in the case of my patient Russ in Chapter 1); dizziness, faintness, nausea, increased pulse rate, palpitation, chest congestion, sleeplessness, diarrhea, belching, bloating, flatulence, vomiting, stomach distress or cramps, dermatitis, eczema, hives, rash, excessive itching, fatigue, muscle aches, pains, weakness, joint aches, swelling ankles, feet, and hands, arthritis, persistent and frequent need to urinate, vaginal discharge, abnormal hunger, anxiety crying jags, irritability, depression, mental slowness, hyperactivity, learning disabilities, difficulty in concentrating and remembering.

Despite even a three-month period of abstinence, certain foods remain staunchly allergenic ("fixed" as Dr. Rinkel puts it). "Milk and wheat are two allergens it is almost impossible to overcome," says Dr. Braly, based on several thousand case studies of patients.

One of my patients with both of these allergies asked my help in substituting other foods for milk and wheat in his breakfast menu. He liked cooked wheat cereal with milk and whole wheat toast.

I recommended his using soy milk or homemade applesauce (no sugar added) made with plenty of water to supply the needed liquid. Then I suggested oatmeal, rye cereal, millet, barley, or brown rice, all of which proved satisfactory and permitted him to keep from repeating any one cereal more than every fifth day. I also recommended that he or his wife bake two or three loaves of rye, oatmeal, buckwheat, or barley bread at a time, freezing some for future use. Again, this system permitted him to rotate breads.

MULTI-INGREDIENT FOODS: POSSIBLE CULPRITS

Like Dr. Braly, I warn my patients against using multi-ingredient food products—for instance, salad dressings that have many ingredients, most commercial breads, and catsup, among others. These products can subtly upset an otherwise non-allergenic diet. (Read the labels, if you insist on using such foods!)

Why not make yourself a simple salad dressing with oil and vinegar? In selecting an oil, make sure that you are not sensitive or allergic to the one you pick: olive, sunflower, or safflower. Lemon or mint is a refreshing addition to vegetable or fruit salads. Again, check them out, too, to make sure you're not allergic to them.

On the hazards of multi-ingredient foods, Dr. Braly warns

against the danger of hidden allergens. Assume for the sake of illustration that you're allergic to corn and products derived from it. Are you aware that you experience corn ingredients in many products daily? Envelopes, stamps, stickers, adhesives, ales, aspirin, bacon, pie crusts, cakes, candies, catsup, milk in paper cartons, oleo, preserves, salad dressings, sandwich spreads, deep fat frying mixtures, whole grain crackers, chewing gum, cured hams, ice cream, sausage, creamed soups, soy bean milk, syrups, vanilla, and distilled vinegar all contain corn ingredients.

With so many hidden hazards, is it possible to avoid food allergens and unpleasant accompanying symptoms and the risk of gaining or retaining unwanted, excess weight?

Yes. Some of my patients have managed to do it with a little coaching. However, a clinical ecologist can help make your efforts more methodical and far more successful and rewarding to you. He or she can help make sure that you aren't overlooking certain hidden allergens—not only in your food, but in your work and home environments.

THE BRALY GROUND RULES

However, if you decide to fly solo, you might want to consider Dr. Braly's guidelines for conquering or minimizing food allergies:

1. Use food rotation—no food consumed more than every five days.

2. Keep your nutritional intake at peak values, including vitamin-mineral supplements, pancreatic enzymes, amino acids, sometimes acid-buffering compounds (many allergic individuals are hyperacidic) and, for a small minority, hydrochloric acid.

3. Exercise daily.

4. Get sufficient rest.

5. Reduce all forms of stress, particularly psychological.

6. Eliminate CATS (Pet lovers, relax! CATS are caffeine, alcohol, tobacco, and sugar).

It takes time, thought, effort, planning, and money to re-place your usual diet to eliminate allergens. Yet it pays off in health, well-being, and weight loss.

Dr. Braly sums up the reasons people in growing numbers are doing it. "They're sick and tired of being sick and tired."

Right. And they're also sick and tired of being overweight!

6 | Stress, Adrenal Glands, and Weight Loss

If you want to control your weight, rather than let it control you—and live longer and better, too—give your adrenal glands tender, loving care.

From time to time, various physical, emotional, and mental stressors activate your two tiny, yellow adrenal glands, which fit like caps on top of your kidneys. However, this is business as usual, and such intermittent stimuli only help to keep them working properly. At the opposite pole are regularly repeated, persistent, and long-enduring stressors, or single devastating ones, that deplete your supply of hard-earned hormones. What happens is much like keeping your car's starter churning away when ignition fails and draining your storage battery. Over the long years, your adrenal glands may wear out and, like your battery, no longer can be recharged.

You can preserve these precious glands with TLC but, first, you must be able to recognize your most severe and repetitive stressors before you can avoid or minimize them.

On the surface, this sounds easy, but many stressors, particularly emotional ones, are subtle. Commonly I find that many patients are not even aware that they are under severe stress, even though they complain of jitteriness, anxiety, depression, and overeating.

SIGNS OF STRESS

The following are telltale signs of stress. You may experience some of them.

If you have at least seven of the twenty-two, you are very likely overstressed:

1. Cold hands (despite normal thyroid gland function or thyroid supplementation to make it normal).

2. Eyestrain (frequent nervous blinking).

3. Gritting teeth.

4. Frequent headaches (symptomatic of numerous medical conditions).

5. High blood pressure.

6. Irregular or shallow breathing.

7. Easy irritability.

8. Nervous jittering of a knee or knees when seated.

9. Frequent tapping of fingers.

10. Increase of appetite or sharp decrease.

11. Loss of sense of humor.

12. Loss of interest in sex.

13. Inability to sleep or frequent waking from sleep.

14. Oversleeping.

15. Stomach upset.

16. Difficulty in thinking.

17. Excessive drinking.

18. Excessive smoking.

19. Excessive use of tranquilizers.

20. Tenseness.

21. Non-stop anxiety.

22. Feeling inadequate in the face of circumstances.

IS YOUR JOB A THREAT?

A second way to determine if you are overstressed is to consider your occupation. Is it hazardous? Does it require meeting frequent, rigid deadlines? Are you responsible for the lives of others? Is your job threatened by mechanization, robotics, computers, or other advanced technology?

If more than one of the above applies, you are probably job-stressed.

Cary L. Cooper, professor of organizational psychology, Department of Management Sciences, at the University of Manchester (England) Institute of Science and Technology, an international authority on occupational stress, conducted with six associates a study for *The British Sunday Times* to determine the most stressful occupations from the standpoint of the incidence of alcoholism, heart attacks, heavy smoking, nervous breakdowns, divorces, and related factors. Here are the ratings of occupations in descending order (from ten to one) of the stress they generate, as related by Dr. Cooper to Jim Scheer in a telephone interview:

Miner	8.3
Police officer	7.7
Construction worker	7.5
Journalist	7.5
Commercial pilot	7.5
Prison officer	7.5
Advertising executive	7.3
Dentist	7.3
Actor	7.2
Politician	7.0
Doctor (medical)	6.8
Tax collector	6.8
Film producer	6.5

Nurse	6.5
Firefighter	6.3
Musician	6.3
Teacher	6.2
Personnel director	6.0
Social worker	6.0
Manager	5.7
Public relations officer	5.8
Sales clerk	5.7
Stockbroker	5.5
Bus driver	5.4
Psychologist	5.2
Publishing executive	5.0
Diplomat	4.8
Farmer	4.8
Soldier	4.7
Veterinarian	4.5
Civil servant	4.4
Accountant	4.3
Engineer	4.3
Real estate broker	4.3
Hairdresser	4.3
Secretary	4.3
Lawyer	4.3
Artist, designer	4.2
Architect	4.0
Optician	4.0
Planner (city, county, state)	4.0
Postman or Postwoman	4.0
Statistician	4.0

Lab technician	3.8
Banker	3.7
Computer operator	3.7
Occupational therapist	3.7
Linguist	3.7
Clergy	3.5
Astronomer	3.4
Nursery school assistant	3.5
Museum worker	2.8
Librarian	2.0

Whatever your work, you can minimize job-related stress by precisely identifying your stressors, then trying to cope with them.

Cooper lists five sources of occupational stress: problems with the work itself, with your role in the company or organization, with your career, with work relationships, and with company or organizational structure and climate.

So far as the job is concerned, you may be troubled by:

1. Poor working conditions (high noise level), intense heat, accident hazards without enough protection, crowded conditions, or clutter;

2. Physical danger, as in police work or fire protection (this stressor responds most readily to taking all available training and using all equipment that make the work safer);

3. Handling hazardous materials;

4. Work overload (too much to do or inability to do the job properly or feeling incapable);

5. Tough schedules, severe time pressure.

Stress also comes from the organization: (1) not understanding your specific role; (2) job conflict (doing work you don't like or think you shouldn't have to do); (3) having responsibility for others.

A career furnishes its own brand of stressors: inability to win promotions, or being over-promoted and suffering feelings of inadequacy and job insecurity.

Relationships, too, may be stressors: negative relations with your boss, subordinates, or co-workers; problems in delegating or taking responsibility.

Organizational structure and climate are additional sources of stress: being left out of the decision-making process; restriction of plans and goals by limited budgets; frustration of dealing with office politics.

Once you identify your stress, you can take remedial action. You can call your boss's attention to it and enlist his or her help in taking correction action. You may have to persist in an inoffensive manner.

If you realize that there are inadequacies or gaps in your knowledge about the work, study to strengthen your weaknesses. You might also try to take a more positive attitude toward job problems. Another alternative is to seek a transfer within the organization or company. If all else fails, you might seek and find another position before resigning from the present one.

Stating that overeating or undereating are common symptoms of stress, Cooper feels that various measures may be of some help.

"Running, sauna, meditation, and biofeedback could all make positive contributions," he says. "By meditation, I don't mean the mumbo-jumbo type, just quiet relaxation. These are useful techniques to help you cope with the symptoms of stress. However, you must grapple with the basics, the underlying problems, because only by doing that will you get rid of the symptoms of stress."

And we must do this to minimize effects of stressors because they contribute directly and indirectly to impaired digestion and assimilation, diminished benefits from food, and a consequent craving for more food than required.

Let's look at what extreme stress does so that we can appreciate what happens even under mild, everyday stress. In "fight or flight" situations, you need every ounce of energy to supply the large muscles for instant, strenuous action. Your heart and lungs accelerate action to draw in extra oxygen and discharge carbon dioxide.

Even your sight and hearing become super-sensitized. Your digestion comes to an abrupt halt to conserve energy, as Dr. Walter Cannon demonstrated many years ago in experiments described in numerous publications.

The problem is that subtle stressors, emotional reactions, have far-reaching consequences. Some of them were covered in a classic *Reader's Digest* article, "The High Cost of Hate."

Hatred, long-held grudges (an unforgiving spirit), anxiety, and fears impair gastrointestinal efficiency, causing poor digestion, absorption, and assimilation of food.

Such a condition is far more serious than merely overeating to appease the body, which knows it is being short-changed of needed nutrients.

The physically inactive suffer especially from hatred, anxieties, and fears, because they do not have an outlet for their response to "fight or flight" situations.

Consequently, their tissues are involved in a biochemical conflict, a ceaseless civil war that, like all such campaigns, exacts payment of war debts. These persons are being depleted of nourishment and energy, while stressful conditions prevent them from efficient nutritional replenishment. The bottom line is that this condition brings on insidious, increased chronic disease even in the prime years, as well as an unconscious tendency to overeat in order to compensate. The resultant added weight imposes another burden on existing heavy and, sometimes, crushing human concerns.

In the previous chapter, we discussed the three distinct stages of stress: alarm, adaptation, and exhaustion responses.

SUPER STRESSORS

Physical stress includes such things as major surgery, severe burns, a serious car accident, chemotherapy, crash diets, fasting, physical immobility, physical exhaustion, animal and snake bites, and infections. Long exposure to intense cold or heat, rarefied air, electric shock or radiation constitutes stress as well.

Examples of extreme emotional stress are: grief over an important loss (the death of a loved one), protracted frustration, depression, mental illness, imprisonment, being fired from a job, retirement, prolonged sickness of a family member, pregnancy, and acute sexual problems.

If one or more of these catastrophes strikes, and your body's adaptation is inadequate, serious illness or even death may result.

In an auto accident, for example, a person could quickly go through the alarm, adaptation, and exhaustion stages. However, it is not uncommon to experience many alarm reactions and adaptations in succession before the stress-handling, glandular system is overwhelmed.

For more than a generation, the Hans Selye model of general stress response was regarded as the accepted description of what happens after a stressor strikes. Selye thought that any stimulus would elicit the same general stress response.

Nobel laureate Julius Axelrod, biochemist at the National Institutes of Mental Health in Bethesda, Md., now feels that the Selye theory may oversimplify what actually happens when one is stressed.[1] Axelrod states that the body doesn't respond generally and uniformly to various stresses. Rather, its defense system is much more finely tuned, reacting to different types of stress in different ways, with a unique neurochemical pathway for each type of response.

THE STRESS SCENARIO

Various hormones in the blood trigger the adrenal glands, and a chemical emergency procedure breaks loose. The adrenal cortex (the outer layer) and the medulla (center) produce hormones. Those from the adrenal cortex sound the alarm. Blood pressure rises dramatically. Proteins from the thymus and lymph glands are converted to sugar for instant energy. Blood sugar rockets upward, and surplus sugar is rushed to the liver, where it is converted into glycogen and stored, ready for rapid change into glucose, if required. Minerals are marshaled out of the bones. Fat is drawn out of its storage areas. Heartbeat and breathing are increased.

All the while, rapidly recruited biochemical raw materials are rushed to the front for use to repair critical areas of tissue. After the emergency, most of the borrowed materials are returned to the lender. This is all part of the alarm reaction.

Should the stress continue, the body will draw frantically on all raw materials available. If the diet is substantial, this emergency borrowing of protein, minerals, fat, and vitamins can be paid back in the post-emergency period with little harm done. However, if stress is unrelenting and nutrition substandard, the storehouse of reserves eventually runs low or out. This is the exhaustion stage. Tissue repairs can't be made, and serious illness often results, with the possible threat of death.[2]

Incessant stress causes the drawing of proteins from the thymus and lymph glands until these glands have shriveled or atrophied. Still the need for protein continues, and the body draws protein wherever it can be found—in the blood plasma, kidneys, liver, and stomach, among other places.

Stomach ulcers result not only from a cannibalizing of proteins from the stomach walls, but also from the great production of hydrochloric acid during stress. Endless stress also may be a causative factor in ulcerative colitis by drawing protein out of the intestinal lining.

Such adaptive self-destruction is also taking place in our bones, from which calcium is removed to satisfy the insatiable appetite of the body's alarm mechanism.

PROTEIN AND VITAMINS TO THE RESCUE

The amount of protein that may be used up in one day of extreme stress equals the protein supplied by four quarts of milk, as measured by the tremendous nitrogen loss in the urine. It has been scientifically demonstrated that when an adequate amount of protein supplement is consumed to meet the body's emergency needs, internal destruction of tissue is stopped.[3]

Extra vitamin A is essential for stressed individuals to keep the adrenal glands from swelling and overproducing cortisone, which can destroy protection-giving lymph cells and shrink the thymus gland, decreasing its effectiveness in the immune system.[4]

A stunning experiment by Dr. Eli Seifter and associates at Albert Einstein Medical College in New York City shows how protective additional vitamin A can be in conditions of devastating stress.[5]

Dr. Seifter's researchers stressed mice without injuring them by placing them in a partial cast to prevent normal movements. Later examination of these animals showed enlargement of their adrenal glands and shrinkage of their thymus—two signs of excessive stress, as indicated by Selye.

Large doses of vitamin A given by the Seifter researchers to another group of similarly stressed mice reduced adrenal enlargement and thymus shrinkage. After the mice were released, their adrenal glands and thymus were restored to normal size by supplementary vitamin A.

Unless optimally supplied with nutrients, our adrenal glands cannot properly protect us from stress. With subnormal nutrition and stress, the entire glandular symphony plays noise, rather than music.

Deprived of pantothenic acid (vitamin B-5) your adrenals shrivel, filling up with dead cellular debris and blood. This limits their ability to produce protective hormones, probably numbering in the hundreds. To sum it up, stress and low intake of pantothenic acid may bring on physical complications and compound effects of additional stress.[6]

Pantothenic acid is an enabler. Cholesterol is the basic material for adrenal, pituitary, and sex hormones. Without sufficient pantothenic acid, these glands cannot rid themselves of used cholesterol and replace it with new. Furthermore, a seemingly minor deficiency of this vitamin greatly reduces the amount of hormones released. A long deprivation of pantothenic acid under protracted stress cannot be made up rapidly even by using liberal amounts of this vitamin. Repair can go on for weeks, and total repair is not always a sure thing. However, if the deficiency has been neither severe nor long, high intake of pantothenic acid can again start the chemical factory producing adrenal hormones overnight.[7]

A grueling experiment demonstrated conclusively how a form of pantothenic acid, calcium pantothenate, made it possible for men to endure physical stress better.[8]

MEN OF ICE

Elaine P. Ralli, M.D., had hardy adult males immerse themselves in icy water for long periods. Tests of body chemistry, made right after their ordeal, revealed extreme stress. Then Dr. Ralli put the men on oral calcium pantothenate for six weeks and once more got them to endure the icy water. This time their tests revealed fewer indications of stress, and at much less intensity. Perhaps the most noteworthy change was the fact that test subjects were not depleted of vitamin C as they had been after the first experiment.

By far, the food supplements and foods richest in pantothenic acid are royal jelly, with 35 mg per 100 grams, and brewer's yeast and torula yeast with 11 and 10 mg per gram, respectively. Others include whole rice (8.9), sunflower seeds (5.5), corn (5), lentils (4.8), egg yolk (4.2), peas (3.6), alfalfa (3.3), wheat (2.2), rye (2.6), eggs (2.3), bee pollen (2.2), and wheat germ (2.1).

Like pantothenic acid, adequate intake of vitamin C reduces damage from stress. In serious deficiency of vitamin C, adrenal glands hemorrhage and sharply reduce hormone production. In certain functions, this vitamin appears to compensate for lack of pantothenic acid. Evidence indicates that vitamin C works to rid us of toxic substances, byproducts of stress. This is why large amounts of vitamin C appear in the urine of individuals under stress.

One hundred and forty-four hospitalized senior patients were handicapped by ceasing of adrenal gland function, even when triggered by ACTH, the pituitary gland hormone that activates the adrenal stress function in normal individuals.[9]

Then they were given 500 mg of vitamin C daily, and the adrenal glands became unusually active again, as measured in both the blood and urine.

Small deficiencies of linoleic acid also depress adrenal hormone production.[10] Best sources in supplements and foods are sesame seeds, soy oil, walnuts, safflower oil, trout, egg yolks, pecans, beans, herring, lamb, sole, and millet.

Similarly, shortages of protein and vitamin B complex—mainly vitamin B-2, pantothenic acid, and choline (another member of the B family)—make it difficult to synthesize enough pituitary hormones to make your adrenal glands work.[11]

No gland has a greater concentration of vitamin E—no part of the body, for that matter—than the pituitary. One of vitamin E's most significant contributions is to keep the pituitary and adrenal hormones from being degraded by oxygen, essential to life but also a contributor to death through oxidation of glands and organs.[12]

MEGA WEIGHT LOSS ANTI-STRESS FORMULA

Here is the formula I use for my heavily stressed patients: between 80 to 120 grams of protein daily from eggs, milk, yogurt or cheese, muscle meats, fish, fowl, and wheat germ. After stress is reduced, protein intake can be cut to 60 grams daily.

The next key ingredients are a minimum of 500 mg of vitamin C, 100 mg of pantothenic acid, and no less than 25 mg of vitamin B-complex with every meal and before going to sleep.

In extreme cases, even super high-powered nutrients can't bail out the depleted adrenal glands. There remains another approach: supplementation with miniscule dosages of cortisone. Before you raise your hands in horror because of the scare stories about cortisone, hear this.

THE OTHER SIDE OF CORTISONE

Once predicted to be a bright, new star in medicine, cortisone never quite equaled its publicity and fell into disrepute because of its horrendous side effects. But most physicians now believe it does not deserve its lowly status.

As pointed out in great detail and with great good sense by William M. Jefferies, M.D., of Cleveland, Ohio, in his book *Safe Uses of Cortisone* (Charles C. Thomas, Publisher):

"Cortisone and hydrocortisone are natural hormones and when properly administered, are as safe as any other naturally produced hormones. In addition to its primary role in response to stress of any type, hydrocortisone has beneficial symptomatic effects in many diseases of humans, but its use has been limited because of fear of harmful side effects that may occur with the pharmacologic dosages that have been customary."[13]

Sluggish adrenal glands can be stimulated by small dosages of hydrocortisone. I prescribe 5 mg four times daily before meals (it is less likely to cause acid indigestion taken at that time) and just before bedtime. My patients have had excellent success with this regimen, which has been tested clinically by Dr. Jefferies for more than thirty years.

I am thankful for Dr. Jefferies's regime and for the nutritional supplementation to cope with the damage caused by stress. However, prevention is the most effective form of treatment.

With few exceptions, damage from stress results from a negative emotional response to stressors, rather than from the stressors themselves. You may not always be able to control what stressors act upon you, but you can usually control your reactions to them.

IMPORTANCE OF STAMINA

Dr. Caroline B. Thomas, of the department of medicine of Johns Hopkins University School of Medicine, studied 1,300 of the university's students over a sixteen-year period, and found that stamina is the secret to coping with physical and emotional stress. What is her definition of stamina?

"The physical or moral strength required to resist or withstand disease, fatigue, or hardship; endurance derived from stamen, 'the thread of life.' "[14]

PATTERN FOR BEATING STRESS

You can minimize or eliminate much of the damage of stress if you follow my ground rules for managing yourself during adversity:

1. Be realistic about goals and the time allowed to reach them. Remember that Superman and Wonder Woman are fictional characters.

2. Don't store up hurts. Let others know if they have let you down, embarrassed, or hurt you.

3. Learn to relax, first by tensing every part of your body progressively, then letting go.

4. Don't be all things to all people. This builds stress. Be yourself. Express that wonderful uniqueness inside you.

5. Keep a positive outlook. This will make you feel and be happier.

6. You won't always win. No one does. So don't condemn yourself if you lose occasionally. Spend time constructively in finding new approaches to your objectives.

7. Preserve your self-esteem. Don't let it falter if you have a failure. Admit to yourself: "I have failed." Never admit, "I am a failure."

8. Don't try to relax by playing highly competitive athletic games such as tennis, handball, or volleyball. Life is competitive enough. Choose restful pursuits: gardening, listening to soothing music, walking through the countryside or on the beach, or following a relaxing hobby that puts you into neutral gear.

9. Plan your work day. Even if you don't complete everything, at least you will have the guidance and security of a pattern to follow.

10. Don't let a mountain of work on your desk intimidate you. Give a priority to every task in order of importance and deadline and take one job at a time—as you do when the workload is smaller.

11. Don't play the "what if?" game about possible threatening events of the distant future. (Most of them won't happen.) This is borrowing trouble. Take one day at a time.

12. Don't magnify problems through your fears. Be realistic about them.

13. Refrain from taking "working vacations." Take vacationing vacations. Rest and restore yourself with a change of pace and a change of place, if possible.

14. Don't always insist that you're right—even when you are. The battle creates tension that may make it worthwhile to come in second sometimes.

15. Get outside yourself, your preoccupations, and your problems by helping others.

16. Develop a group of supportive persons. You build confidence and relieve stress by belonging.

17. Talk out your problems, fears, and anxieties with trusted associates, friends, or relatives. You'll feel better and reinforced.

18. Create islands of relaxation several times a day—during breaks and at lunchtime. Review fun vacations you have taken and other times of joy and satisfaction.

19. Keeping super-high expectations for yourself and others under all conditions only leads to disappointment and frustration. Be understanding and realistic. No one is at his or her best at all times.

20. Work off frustration and tension with low-key sports activities or exercise. Dissipate stress by beating up on a punching bag or a pillow. Jump rope, take a brisk walk, or jog.

21. Don't dwell on mistakes or misfortunes. Learn from them and move ahead.

These suggestions will help you handle stress before it can manhandle you.

Above all, remember Dr. Cooper's recommendation. Whenever possible, deal with the basic cause of stress, rather than with the symptoms.

And don't forget, people under stress tend to undereat or overeat. The latter brings on overweight, sometimes obesity. Extra pounds are an added stress, something nobody needs.

7 | Heavy Metals, Heavy People

Still other stressors, heavy metals, are so notorious as ravagers of good health and silent assassins that you rarely, if ever, hear that they can help you put on and keep unwanted weight.

This is why I didn't initially suspect that metal intoxication was the basic problem of my new patient, Evelyn, a short, plump, thirty-five-year-old homemaker, whose major complaints were depression, intermittent pain in the liver area, low blood sugar, and overweight.

"I'm in a black depression, and the only thing that seems to help is food," she told me. "I eat non-stop."

Probing questions revealed that her diet was about 70 percent carbohydrate and the rest fats and proteins. As she lay on the table and I touched her liver, she cried out in pain. The liver was definitely enlarged and inflamed.

I wondered if fatty degeneration was beginning. Could Evelyn be a secret alcoholic? When I asked if she drank alcohol, she responded directly and sincerely, "Hardly ever."

Her low-protein diet, including no choline or methionine and little vitamin C, appeared to be worsening a liver disorder, which probably also accounted for her low blood sugar and ravenous appetite.

Although the liver is an incredible organ with amazing regenerative power, I was fearful about her, because liver inflammation and swelling often lead to fatty degeneration, then to cirrhosis.

Was some environmental poison stressing her liver? I questioned her about possible exposure to chemicals, drugs, insecticides, weed-killers, or cleaning solvents such as carbon tetrachloride. Finally, she zeroed in on something that seemed helpful. For the past ten years she had lived in an apartment on a heavily traveled corner on the edge of the city's commercial area.

"The apartment is right behind a big service station," she told me.

Lightning couldn't have hit me harder. Facts of a study made in Switzerland some years before filled my mind. It had been found that various types of cancer—lung and liver, among others—were almost epidemic in houses bordering a major highway bisecting the town.

The cancer incidence was almost negligible in residents whose houses were several hundred yards from the road. The study's conclusion was that car exhaust, laden with lead, was the primary cause.

Although little leaded gasoline is now sold in the United States, Evelyn apparently had breathed in more lead than she needed. A hair analysis made by a reliable laboratory confirmed my suspicion, with an alarmingly high reading of lead.

HOW TO LESSEN LEAD LOAD

I recommended that she move into an apartment in a residential area away from heavy street traffic. Then I put her on a diet high in complex protein—80 grams a day—with 5,000 units of vitamin C, 50 mg of B-complex, 25,000 I.U. of vitamin A, 600 I.U. of vitamin E, and lecithin for its choline and methionine. I insisted that she desist from all junk food.

On her new regime, she was feeling better at her next appointment a week later. Her liver hardly pained her. Her appetite was a little less demanding, and she felt less depressed.

Five weeks after our first meeting, she found a new apartment in a residential area and in the right rental bracket. Meanwhile the new diet was treating her liver properly, and the vitamin

C was transporting the lead out. The liver was now less tender and slightly smaller.

Two months later when I saw her again, she had lost fourteen pounds. After another two months, she was "feeling great" and proud that another eight pounds had melted away.

Some persons in the United States tend to pooh-pooh the lead problem, saying "Almost all gasoline sold today is non-leaded, so there's no problem."

On the contrary, there is a problem—a serious one. Several surveys have pointed out that we have a tremendous lead burden—500 times more than our ancestors of two generations ago—and that all sorts of medical problems arise from this, particularly high blood pressure even when exposure to lead is at low levels.

Aware of the gravity of this situation, a research organization, the Olive W. Garvey Center for the Improvement of Human Functioning, Inc., in Wichita, Kansas, is experimenting to find a way to solve the problem.

The center is using ethylene-diamine-tetra-acetic acid (EDTA) to bind with the lead and other heavy metals and usher them out of the body in the urine. The purpose is to determine whether lead removal from hypertensive test subjects really will lower elevated blood pressure.

SOURCES OF LEAD

A question patients often ask me is, "If there's so much lead around, where is it coming from?"

Much of it is already here, from the many years autos have spread pollution from leaded fuel. It has settled on the ground, in streams, and on drinking-water reservoirs. Rain has carried it into the soil, where vegetables, grains, grasses for cattle, and trees pick it up and incorporate it into our food supply. Almost everything we eat has at least traces of lead.

Automobile exhaust is just one of many sources. Lead arsenate is another. This is a combination of lead and arsenic with which fruit trees still are sprayed. Some of it ends up on the fruit itself. As much as 1,800 pounds are sprayed on an acre of land within a ten-year period.

Lead arsenate also is sometimes sprayed on tobacco as an insecticide, offering lead pollution to the smoker and everyone in his or her environment.

How else do we get our daily lead?

Some pencils chewed upon by children and adults are still coated with lead-based paint. Lead leaches into our food from earthenware plates whose lead glaze is fixed at too-low temperatures. It enters our digestive tract from toothpaste in lead tubes, and from sealants for metal cans containing foods and beverages (another good reason for eating fresh foods).

Pet foods eaten by some impoverished individuals contain meats from animal organs, a favorite accumulation depot for lead. One hundred seventy grams (six ounces) of pet food daily could add as much as 1.19 mg of lead to the diet of a pet or person. According to Carl C. Pfeiffer, Ph.D., M.D., this is four times the amount that could be toxic to children.[1]

Additionally, people buy and use fresh organ meat as sausage and sandwich spread. These are heavy on lead—especially liverwurst.

Two researchers, Hankin and Heichel, of the Connecticut Agricultural Experiment Station, analyzed seven different brands of liverwurst sold in stores and found their lead content to be from 1.8 to 7.6 parts per million. Even a total of 113 grams (four ounces) eaten daily by human beings could mean an intake of lead from 0.20 to 0.86 mg. This is a range of 0.6 to 2.9 times the amount of lead that could be poisonous to children.[2]

Fresh pork liver samples revealed lead levels as high as 5.6 parts per million. Beef and turkey livers registered even higher amounts: 7.6 ppm and 10 ppm, respectively. (There goes my turkey giblet gravy!) Pfeiffer mentions pork liver as a double threat; it contains not only lead but copper, another toxic heavy metal. Farmers often add copper sulphate to fodder for hogs, to make them gain weight faster. Excessive copper also helps us gain and retain weight, as it poisons us. Copper is a necessary nutrient, but only in amounts up to five mg daily. In excess, it is a zinc antagonist. Copper also oxidizes vitamin C. Pfeiffer notes that high intake of copper may even contribute to developing schizophrenia.

I warn my patients to beware of taking excessive mineral supplements and to stay near the Recommended Daily Allowance (RDA). Individuals who overdo mineral supplements can seriously harm themselves. Their philosophy seems to be, "If a little bit does me some good, a lot more will do me a lot more good."

Sorry, but you're wrong! While there is often a broad range of tolerance for using vitamin supplements, this is not generally true with minerals.

A story told to me by a Massachusetts physician at a medical convention about a decade ago drives home this point better than any warning. (The story was later written up in several medical journals, so it was amply verified.)

THE GREEN HAIR EPIDEMIC

An epidemic of green hair broke out in the city of Framingham. It was particularly conspicuous among the blond girls at Framingham State College.

The cause? The city's water supply, as scientific sleuthing eventually disclosed. Sodium fluoride had recently been introduced into the drinking water to fight dental cavities, and it did much more than that. Fluoride made the water more acid, and the acid leached copper out of the pipes.

As mentioned earlier, copper is a zinc antagonist. This fact is of special significance, because zinc performs numerous key body functions. Zinc is essential to the healing process and teams with vitamin A in numerous biochemical tasks. It contributes to the operation of more than a dozen critical enzymes and, of major importance to weight control, it is vitally necessary in synthesizing of insulin, affecting both hypoglycemia and diabetes.

Zinc and copper compete for the same intestinal absorption site. When a disproportionate amount of copper is ingested, the copper can interfere with zinc absorption.

When excessive zinc is taken in, copper is blocked from absorption.

CADMIUM CAN MAKE YOU GAIN

Cadmium, unlike copper and zinc, is not required in human nutrition—in fact, it is toxic—and yet it invades the body, settling in the liver and kidneys. Cadmium can cause dysfunction of the blood-sugar economy and, in this way, contribute to accumulation of excess weight.

In the manner of copper, cadmium can enter the body when soft water leaches it from pipes. Fortunately, it is difficult to absorb from the diet. But it isn't so difficult to absorb from inhaling cigarette smoke, big city air pollution, and air near a zinc refinery.

Once in the body, cadmium can cause pulmonary emphysema, anemia, proteinuria, and amino aciduria, along with toxic effects in the liver and kidneys. And it can remain in the body for decades. Cadmium not only works to undermine the health of cigarette smokers but also that of nonsmokers exposed to their smoke.[3]

Abundant dietary calcium—at least 1,000 mg daily—is one of your best allies against cadmium and lead. Calcium may be able to prevent lead-related atherosclerosis of the aorta and high blood pressure, as demonstrated in rat experiments.[4]

Another heavy metal that threatens us from various sources is mercury, a silvery, highly toxic liquid metal, which, like cadmium, is often absorbed by inhalation.

SLOW POISONING FROM MERCURY

Salts of mercury are widespread in the environment—in agriculture, industry, and medicine—so it is possible to be poisoned slowly from it in various environments.

A common place for exposure is the dentist's office, where mercury is combined with silver—35 to 50 percent—as an amalgam filling for teeth.

Individuals who have a mouthful of these fillings may be suffering from a degree of mercury toxicity as acids gradually leech it into the mouth and down the digestive tract.

Mercury's sabotage is slow and subtle in some instances, fast and obvious in others. Its most devastating harm comes from weakening the structure of protein and making it useless.[5] Such destruction is more far-reaching and serious than it may sound. Remember that antibodies, enzymes, hemoglobin, and hormones are largely composed of protein.

Most vulnerable to mercury's effects are persons who mine it and those who have been exposed to it for long periods: dentists and others who work in dentists' offices. A growing group of conscientious and responsible dentists is concerned about installing mercury-containing fillings in the mouths of patients, and also about the hazards of handling and storing mercury.

Hal Huggins, D.D.S., of Colorado Springs, Colorado, cites cases of 200 patients who suffered from an assortment of medical disorders associated with amalgam fillings and who recovered when the fillings were replaced with harmless nonmetallic substances.

However, the American Dental Association (ADA) takes the stance that the problem has been blown out of all proportion and that no substantial research indicts amalgam fillings.

Despite this position, it has been shown that even minute amounts of mercury—similar to that leeched from fillings—can cause illness. Of five cases of mercury poisoning in infants mentioned in the *British Medical Journal*, four were caused by the same product.[6]

When babies were brought to the hospital with extreme symptoms—violent diarrhea and vomiting as well as serious and generalized edema (tissue swelling)—doctors were puzzled as to the cause. Then they discovered that one of the children was discharging inordinate amounts of mercury in his urine.

Questioning of the parents revealed that teething powder had been given to the infants regularly for three to eighteen months. One of the main ingredients of the powder was calomel, mercurous chloride.

During the late 1970s, Willem H. Khoe, M.D., Ph.D., who practices preventive medicine in Las Vegas, Nevada, studied the issue of amalgam fillings in almost 100 years of medical journals. He found that most of the research revealed that mercury fillings were harmful to the health.

REVEALING RESEARCH

On the basis of medical literature, David W. Eggleston, D.D.S., suspected that amalgam fillings depress the immune system. Dr. Eggleston, clinical associate professor of the Department of Restorative Dentistry at the University of Southern California, who has a private practice in Newport Beach, California, launched a research project in 1983 to investigate his premise.

He enlisted test subjects who, for the benefit of mankind and possible benefit to themselves, would submit to having all amalgam fillings removed and replaced with nontoxic fillings.

Jim Scheer, my collaborator, participated in Eggleston's preliminary study, offering blood samples for analysis before the experiment and after removal of amalgam fillings.

At the experiment's end, the number of his T-lymphocite cells, in ratio to total lymphocyte cells, rose by more than 30 percent, an appreciable strengthening of his immune function.

A few words about lymphocytes will offer a frame of reference for appreciating the significance of this improvement.

White blood cells called lymphocytes are produced in lymph glands. Those that pass through the thymus gland, the master gland of the immune system, are changed to T-lymphocytes. As we add years, the thymus gland shrinks and reduces its production of hormones. This is a major reason that so much cancer occurs later in life, and that autoimmune disorders are so prevalent then. In the latter conditions, the defender cells attack the body they are supposed to defend.

In the arsenal of a strong immune system, 70 to 86 percent of lymphocytes are T-lymphocytes, but a range of 53 to 86 percent is regarded as normal. Two major kinds of T-cells have been discovered: the helper T-lymphocytes (called T-4 cells) and suppressor lymphocytes (called T-8 cells).

The helper T-lymphocytes identify and label harmful organisms, cancer cells, and foreign bodies. Unless the T-4 lymphocytes label these invaders, the macrophages and other white blood cells won't attack and destroy them.

Obviously, then, if the helper cells don't work properly or if their army is too small, the immune system militia is depressed and conceivably could be outnumbered and immobilized by the enemy.

Acquired immune deficiency syndrome (AIDS) is an extreme example of how the body can be devastated by Kaposi's Sarcoma and infections because there are too few or too few capable helper lymphocytes.

The other mentioned thymus-modified cells, the suppressor T-8 lymphocytes, balance the action of the macrophages and other white blood cells to keep them from attacking normal body cells. To maintain the delicate balance of the T-4 and T-8 cells, their ratio should be between 1.8 to 1 to 2 to 1, respectively.

If the ratio is below the first figure or above the latter, the person may be vulnerable to autoimmune disease—glomerulonephritis (medical gibberish for damage to the infinitesimal kidney filtering units), hemolytic anemia, inflammatory bowel disease, multiple sclerosis, severe atopic eczema and, among others, systemic lupus erythematosus (which affects skin and organs), and Hashimotos Autoimmune Thyroiditis.

Various studies have shown that T-lymphocyte percent of total lymphocytes varies by no more than 10 percent. Rarely does it fluctuate by more than 5 percent in an eight-week period.

MERCURY VERSUS THE IMMUNE SYSTEM

Within this frame of reference, here is one of Dr. Eggleston's most fascinating cases.[7]

A twenty-one-year-old symptomless white woman with no significant medical history was found to have seven amalgam fillings and one dental cavity in the making. Before the amalgam was removed, her reading of T-lymphocytes was 47 percent. After the amalgam was removed and replaced with provisional fillings, 73 percent of her lymphocytes were T-lymphocytes—an increase of 53.3 percent.

For the sake of research, this patient permitted Dr. Eggleston to reinsert four amalgam fillings. This change made the percentage of T-lymphocytes drop from 73 percent to 55 percent—a decrease of 24.7 percent.

After the amalgam and provisional restoration were removed and replaced with eight gold fillings, 72 percent of her lymphocytes were T-lymphocytes—up from 55 percent, a gain of 30.9 percent.

Dr. Eggleston had similar results with two other patients.

Evidence cited throughout this chapter indicates that heavy metals can, indeed, affect the liver, disturb the balance of blood sugar, and even depress the immune system.

As ably demonstrated in the best-seller, *Dr. Berger's Immune Power Diet*, by Stuart Berger, M.D., of New York City, immune system strength must be maintained in order for us to keep our weight under control.

8 | The Immune Connection

Until *Dr. Berger's Immune Power Diet* became a smashing best-seller, few individuals except specialized medical researchers realized that the immune system had any bearing on overweight.

Although, unlike Dr. Berger, I do not have 3,000 case histories in my files that show this relationship, I have enough to convince me that he is right and that research to come will bear him out.

My case histories indicate that there is a correlation between being overweight or obese and a decline in efficient function of the immune system, contributing to more weight gain and, consequently, more loss in immune system efficiency.

Every pound of fat that you add makes losing weight that much harder. To put it simply, the vicious cycle becomes even more vicious. And every additional pound makes you an easier target for the common cold (an uncommon inconvenience), the flu, bronchitis, asthma, pleurisy, and many other illnesses, courtesy of germs and viruses: cardiovascular disease, diabetes, and cancer.

Although the subject will be covered in more detail later, let me say that the overweight and grossly overweight are not only sick more often than normal-weight persons but, usually, for longer periods. Carrying around their burdens of fat, they are prone to easy fatigue, low energy and stamina, and more depression, which intensifies with added poundage.

Despite the fact that all returns are not in yet, overweight seems to stress the thymus, the immune system's master gland, and to help accelerate its degeneration.

Galen, whose writings in experimental physiology, anatomy, and therapy influenced the practice of medicine for 1,400 years, gave this gland the name thymus because it resembled the flowering thyme, a fragrant herb.

Situated in the upper chest just below the throat, the thymus begins degenerating early—when we are about fourteen years old. The decline and fall of the thymus is partly due to nature and partly due to how we treat it. Rapid decline is associated with more rapid aging and greater susceptibility to illness and degenerative diseases.

YOUR THYMUS GLAND MAY BE THREATENED

Due to the stresses of life (including overweight), improper eating, and dietary deficiencies, we hurry the deterioration of the thymus gland.

It is chilling to see what food allergens can do to white blood cells, important members of the immune-system army. Peering through a high-powered microscope, I have seen an incredible sight: food allergens in a drop of a patient's blood attacking these cells, changing their shape, and actually causing them to explode.

Multiplying this effect by a number of food allergens, you can imagine how such a stress can weaken the immune system. Add to this the fluid retention common to persons with food sensitivities, allergy, and fat storage, and you have an additional stress—leaving you wide open to infectious diseases and degenerative disorders, plus discouragement and the tendency to overeat.

One of my new patients whom I'll call Kay illustrated this point. If there were disease germs and viruses around, they homed in on Kay, who was about thirty-four pounds over her ideal weight. She had had an unbelievable succession of illnesses: colds, flu, cystitis (bladder infection), bronchitis, asthma, colitis, swollen ankles, feet, and hands, and then a reprise of cystitis and flu.

On the basis of her repeated infections—particularly of the respiratory tract—I suspected thyroid insufficiency. However, results of the Barnes Basal Temperature Test were normal, and she showed no confirming symptoms and history.

One test after another ruled out Candida albicans, adrenal insufficiency, and hypoglycemia, so we narrowed her problem down to food or environmental substance hypersensitivity and a weakened immune system.

Kay had always been sensitive to milk products, which caused intestinal disorder—nausea, flatulence, and occasional griping. At first, she disavowed having had milk products, but it turned out she had a passion for New England clam chowder, which is heavy on milk or cream.

All I did was suggest a seafood restaurant where they served Manhattan clam chowder (the red stuff) and she could take out several pints to store in her freezer.

Eventually, we also found out that she was allergic to corn and products made from it. Eliminating milk and corn products reduced the stress on her immune system, and soon the depressing parade of disorders slowed down. Within six months, it came to a halt.

In the process, Kay lost twenty-one pounds. She is on the way to losing more by systematically tracking down and cutting out other culprit foods and strengthening her immune system in the process.

SOLVING A BAFFLING MYSTERY

One of my most puzzling cases concerned an appreciably overweight salesman for a printing company. In work that demanded high energy, enthusiasm, and persistence, Lon could hardly drag himself from appointment to appointment. His enthusiasm was all in the past tense. His sales sagged like his energy level and endurance. Never ill before, Lon had gone through a series of infections—ear, nose, throat, and urinary tract. It seemed that low thyroid function could be the cause. However, the Barnes Basal Temperature Test and his medical history, or lack of it, ruled that out.

Could it be adrenal exhaustion? Lab tests failed to support my suspicion.

Perhaps anxiety over his health, flagging sales, customer rejection, declining self-esteem, fear of losing his position, and overweight were over-stressing his immune system. If not, why would he be fighting infection after infection?

When a patient's health, livelihood, and self-esteem are threatened, I can't get the problem out of my mind. My office work becomes my homework. Lon's was one of those day-and-night cases. Several nights later, I woke from a fitful sleep with what might be a clue.

I remembered having read in a vintage physiology book something that might be helpful. The specific detail eluded me. In my pajamas, I combed every medical book in my home library without finding what I needed.

Earlier than usual, I left home that morning for my Berkeley office without breakfast. After an hour of skimming my medical books, I found what I had half remembered in a book called *Glandular Physiology and Therapy* (Fifth Edition), written by many contributors under the auspices of the Council on Pharmacy and Chemistry of the American Medical Association.

This is the gist of it: The release of immune globulin is under control of the adrenal cortex, and mobilization of antibodies is related to a specific type of resistance. When the level of adrenal hormone of the body is raised by the taking of a cortical extract, corticotropin or by *various stresses* (the emphasis is mine) lymphocyte cells formed in the lymph glands—important to the making of antibodies—are dissolved. However, this finding was not consistent with those of other researchers.

Yet the book had given me a clue. Stress could be doing to Lon's lymphocytes what milk and corn had been doing to Kay's white blood cells!

During my next interview with Lon, I put him on six small meals a day, the same number of calories as he had been eating in three meals, but with a higher protein content. I also put him on the anti-stress formula described in Chapter 6 and talked him into a mild, regular exercise program—walking for twenty minutes twice daily to help break tension, improve his blood circulation, and stimulate his lymph glands.

Lon even went along with trying to cry when alone to relieve stress, the technique described by biochemist Dr. William Frey, of St. Paul Ramsey Medical Center of St. Paul, Minnesota.

Maybe macho men don't cry and real men don't eat quiche, but I convinced him that overly stressed men—or women—who want to get well should cry if necessary.

This multi-pronged approach slowly changed Lon's condition for the better. With each week's office visit, he improved in energy and endurance and lost a half pound to a pound and one-half. Best of all, he no longer had infections. His self-esteem and enthusiasm soon returned.

The last time I saw him, he confided, "Doctor, a few years ago, I was the company's salesman of the year. I'm going to be that again."

THE ZINC DEFICIENCY

Sheila's story was a little different. The owner of a small dress shop, she found herself slowly and progressively moving from a size 10 dress to a size 12 and then a 14. Along with her depressing weight gain came sluggishness and pessimism. Her once trim figure really needed to be trimmed down, and no diet or exercise regime seemed to help.

During her first office visit, I learned she had discovered that her husband of ten years was carrying on extramarital sex. She cried uncontrollably for several minutes.

As with Kay and Lon, I suspected that hypothyroidism or adrenal exhaustion was the underlying cause of Sheila's problem. The shock (stress) of her husband's affair, coupled with her inexplicable weight gain—another underminer of confidence—might be enough to tax her adrenal glands.

However, we were soon able to rule out that, hypothyroidism, and Candida albicans. Sheila's first appointment had been so filled with her anxiety, stress, and the marital problem that I had only cursorily examined her complete diet history. Now I noted that she was an on-again/off-again vegetarian. To her credit, she took a vitamin B-12 supplement when on vegetables and fruits. During her off periods, she binged on junk food.

It occurred to me that she was very likely short-changing her body of the trace mineral zinc, a main raw material for the thymus gland. It would have been necessary for her to eat several heads of lettuce, a head of cabbage, a head of cauliflower, a bunch of carrots, a pound of squash, four large tomatoes, and several turnips to get her daily allowance of zinc: 15 to 25 mg.

Assured that she favored vegetarianism, I persuaded her to eat more oatmeal, one of the most zinc-rich cereals, along with whole-grain rye and wheat with a few tablespoons of wheat germ added and, of course, milk. I also persuaded her to eat two eggs a day, since there was no history of hypercholesterolemia in her family and her cholesterol level and ratio of high-density lipoproteins to low-density lipoproteins were in the normal range.

Within six months of her new regime, Sheila became the Sheila of old, regained her fire, and gradually lost weight by one dress size. She was still shedding weight when I last saw her.

These three cases and several score more since then have convinced me that the immune system has more to do with the body than to defend it against enemies within. In ways not yet clearly understood, the immune system influences the storing of fat or losing it, depending upon its efficiency.

And of paramount importance to immune system efficiency is an active thymus gland. Several studies have established that sufficient intake of zinc can stimulate a tired or aging thymus gland.

In one research project, test subjects deficient in zinc proved to be highly susceptible to infection. However, when sufficient zinc was added, this tendency decreased.

Zinc has a profound effect on immune responses in individual cells and in body fluids—blood and lymph. One experiment demonstrated that impaired cell immune function returned to normal in three weeks of zinc intake at 22.7 mg daily.[1]

In studies of children and animals, it was found that zinc deficiency can cause the thymus gland to atrophy. In comparison, the thymus shrinks more than any other gland because of zinc shortage. Researchers in Jamaica checked the size of eight children's thymus glands by chest radiography prior to, during, and after supplementation with zinc at 2 mg per kilogram of body weight for ten days. All children showed growth in thymus size at experiment's end.[2]

In a controlled test, groups of patients with a severe zinc deficiency developed T-cell abnormality. Following twelve days of intravenous zinc supplementation at 12 mg per day, their T-cell function rose impressively to 221 percent and 139 percent above that of controls.[3]

COMEBACK OF THE THYMUS IN SENIORS

Several experiments show that atrophy of the thymus—even among the elderly—is not necessarily a natural part of the aging process. This may be due particularly to a deficiency of zinc, and of protein, vitamins, and other minerals.

Only a month of oral zinc sulphite supplementation improved the immune response of fifteen seventy-year-old patients. T-lymphocyte cell numbers were increased, and immunoglobulin and antibody response to a vaccine were vastly improved by zinc supplementation.[4]

In still another study, zinc deficiency was shown to contribute to the suppression of the immune function in persons under severe stress such as bereavement.[5]

Zinc teams with vitamin A in many biochemical functions. As we showed in Chapter six, the research of Dr. Eli Seifter of Albert Einstein Medical College revealed how vitamin A protects the thymus gland from shrinkage under stress and helps restore it to normal size after stress is eliminated.

Still another nutrient, fat-soluble vitamin E, makes an important contribution to immune-system effectiveness when taken with the trace mineral selenium. Antibodies are boosted considerably.[6]

LIPOTROPICS STIMULATE THE IMMUNE SYSTEM

And don't forget the lipotropics when considering your thymus. What are lipotropics? Substances that prevent excessive fat from collecting in the liver: betaine, a vitaminlike food fraction found in beets; choline, a B-complex vitamin, mostly richly present in soy lecithin and egg yolks, as well as in lentils, split peas, rice, eggs, and wheat germ; inositol, another B-complex vitamin most abundant in soy lecithin and also in rice, wheat germ, lentils, and barley; and methionine, an essential amino acid most abundantly found in eggs.

Lipotropics stimulate the production of antibodies and the growth and aggressiveness of phagocytes, protective "Pac-Man"-type cells that encompass and destroy invading bacteria, viruses, and abnormal or foreign tissue.[7] They also detoxify the liver and spur its production of lecithin, a substance that emulsifies bubbles of cholesterol and fat in the bloodstream to smaller, less potentially harmful units.

How do these food fractions bolster the immune system and help you keep your weight under control? It is impossible to supply all the whys and wherefores at this writing. However, it is within your power to eat the foods and supplements mentioned to reduce the effects of stress on your immune system, the rest of your body and, most important, the structure of your emotional life.

9 | Are You a Victim of High Calorie Emotions?

Married into immense wealth, Marijane was a woman who had everything, including an over-padded body which no longer could fit into wardrobes full of designer clothing.

"Doctor, it's torture to see those beautiful dresses and not be able to wear them," she complained.

A large-framed woman in her early thirties, attractive despite her excess thirty-five pounds, Marijane had come to me in desperation.

"No matter what other doctors proposed, I couldn't lose an ounce," she sighed. "All I think about is food—meals, between-meal snacks, and between snacks snacks."

It turned out that she had gone through the spectrum of tests closely or even remotely related to overweight—checks of organ and gland function, analysis of digestive tract microorganisms, hair analysis, a six-hour glucose tolerance test, and a comprehensive review of food intake to determine diet insufficiencies.

"I checked out perfectly in every respect but diet, and no one had to tell me I'm heavy on refined carbohydrates."

When the Barnes Basal Temperature Test turned out to be normal, I asked if her problems were emotional. She was skeptical about that.

I cited findings by Dr. Walter Hamburger, professor of psychiatry at Rochester University, who had discovered four types of overeating caused by emotions:

1. In response to nonspecific emotional tensions;

2. To compensate for intolerable life situations;

3. As a sign of hidden emotional illness, particularly as an expression of hysteria;

4. As a food addiction.[1]

UNDERMINING EMOTIONS

Then I mentioned that many psychologists think that unless the emotional basis for overeating is pulled out by the roots and examined, it is impossible to treat overweight and obesity with complete effectiveness.

Dr. Stanley Schachter had stated that some emotional overeating is caused by patients not being able to differentiate between actual hunger feelings and urges to eat motivated by anxiety. Anxious persons may eat to relieve anxiety, rather than to assuage hunger, according to Schachter.[2]

Marijane seemed to be relating these findings to her own case, so I continued. I mentioned that some years earlier, the U.S. Public Health Service had sponsored a well-designed, three-year study on personality and emotions related to overweight.

Drs. Benjamin Kotkov, Stanley S. Kanter, and Joseph Rosenthal at the Boston Dispensary of the New England Medical Center had questioned and tested 135 overweight women and a control group of 80 normal-weight women. They had used multiple psychological techniques to uncover revealing emotional characteristics.[3]

They found that overweight women were far more repressed than those of normal weight—more tense, anxious, and likely to hold anger inside. The latter characteristic often brought on depression. Further, the overweight women tended to be self-preoccupied, neither seeking nor promoting new relationships. They usually did not enjoy social life as much as the women of normal weight, and often were tense and miserable, particularly in meeting new individuals. Some were ill at ease in clothing.

It made no difference if the test subjects were moderately or extremely overweight. They all revealed a somewhat neurotic pattern, regardless of degree of education, I.Q., or whether married or single.

Since this landmark study, many authorities have found that numerous and varied emotional traits, over and above those already mentioned, had motivated individuals to overeat—for example, working year after year in a job they hate, frustration at the inability to progress in a career, or boredom.

"*Boredom!* That's it for me," Marijane cried out. "I'm so bored at having whatever I want whenever I want it, at hosting meaningless parties or attending them, so bored that my life is without meaning that I could scream. I don't, because millions of individuals would love to be in my Guccis."

After we sorted everything out, I recommended that Marijane find a civic project that would give her life a goal, purpose, and direction.

Several weeks later, Marijane had found her niche: planning and implementing a project to create livable quarters for street people. She's too busy with an excellent cause to be bored or to think much about herself. Often, she's too busy to remember to eat.

After a few more months passed, Marijane was losing weight by more than a pound a week and had shed 16 pounds.

"I'm going to lose 19 more pounds," she told me.

My medical files hold numerous cases of overweight patients who have reversed negative emotional characteristics and lost significant poundage. These cases illustrate that certain emotions can indeed undermine the best of intentions to lose weight. I call them high-calorie emotions because they underlie high-calorie intake.

Not long after the solution of Marijane's case, I was rereading *The Stress of Life*, the fine book by Dr. Hans Selye, which covers his stress theory. In one part, he mentions that individuals who are dissatisfied or bored with their work or their social relations often are driven to find consolation in anything that offers comfort.

Just as circumstances and situations may motivate a person to drink, they also may drive certain individuals to overeat. He calls this diversion "the principle of deviation." Some individuals eat because they have nothing better to do—as with Marijane—or as a substitute for doing something better.

Obesity may be a sign of stress—especially in persons subject to frustrating mental experiences. Selye indicates that obesity compounds the emotional state from which overeating originates, producing even greater stress due to the deformity it causes and the cardiovascular illnesses and diabetes that it encourages.

Overeating not only brings gratification to compensate for emotional abuse felt; it also causes the drawing away of blood from the brain, producing a soothing effect, says Selye.

OUTSIDE STIMULANTS FOR OVEREATING

In their book, *Slim Chance in a Fat World* (Research Press), Richard B. Stuart and Barbara Davis, respected weight-control authorities, theorize that cues to overeat do not come only from outside stimuli (objects and events). They also may come from the inside, from internal reactions such as emotions. Stuart and Davis mention that some psychologists find that the obese often are depressed, and that this emotional state probably triggers overeating.[4]

So does rejection, an experience that often precedes depression. A doctoral dissertation by Edward H. Conrad of New York University describes his unique experiment with 108 undergraduate obese and normal-weight students.[5] Conrad offered a display of several foods to individuals ostensibly working on a market survey, during which they were given false reports that they had received a (1) social rejection, (2) neutral social response, or (3) noteworthy social acceptance.

The grossly overweight individuals who had received notice of rejection ate the most food. The normal weights ate the least food when told of rejection. The accepted (heavyweights and lightweights) ate the next most food. Those who had received a neutral response ate the least food.

This experiment made two clear-cut statements: (1) that emotional conditions influence the eating of both overweight and normal-weight subjects, although in the opposite way when the stimulus is negative and (2) that obese individuals do not tend to eat large quantities of food unless in a state of aroused emotions. A related study by J. Rodin, P. Herman, and S. Schachter reveals that, although obesity may have an emotional motivation, it can be controlled by manipulating environmental conditions and events.[6]

In other words, when emotionally upset, don't walk past the cream puff display in the supermarket bakery. And when emotionally stressed, don't take a cruise, in which food is one of the main attractions, no matter how healthful the sea air may be.

THE BIG THREE DIET DESTROYERS

Especially if you're under negative emotional influences, beware of three types of deprivation that Stuart and Davis connect with overindulgence in food: (1) lack of food (meal skipping), (2) lack of sleep (energy deprivation), and (3) lack of stimulation (resulting from boredom).[7]

Meal skipping will make you feel psychologically indebted to yourself to overeat at your next meal. Poor sleep and fatigue will make you want to compensate by overeating. So will an unstimulated life.

Forty obese persons questioned by Stuart disclosed that eating is not even a highly preferred activity. Ranking ahead of eating were socializing, working, affectionate sexual meetings, and personal nonfood enjoyment.

Stuart believes that this finding offers encouragement to the overweight, since the first four favored activities could displace eating if they commanded the individual's attention and offered positive gratification.

If you want to eat less, Stuart advises you to keep occupied with nonfood pursuits and to avoid boredom at all cost.

A team of researchers, comparing eating habits of normal weights and heavyweights, learned that the normals eat because they're hungry, and the obese eat as a result of emotional states: anger, depression, excitement, happiness, or boredom.[8]

An unusual finding is that boredom triggers eating in both normal *and* heavyweight individuals, write Abramson and Stimson.[9]

Excessive eating in response to emotional states, called "reactive overeating," is usually accompanied by a drastic decrease in physical activity, as with grief or severe depression, states Dr. Albert J. Stunkard, one of the world's foremost authorities on weight control. This combination can defeat any efforts to lose weight.[10]

Emotional states help the start of what Dr. Stunkard calls the "night eating syndrome," heavy eating at a time of least physical activity. In the dark of evening with the day's accumulated fatigue come the worst assaults of depression, for which heavyweights compensate with the bulk of their calories.[11]

A study by Stunkard and H.B. Wolff reveals another fascinating fact about emotional conditions and weight gain, particularly depression. There are drastic changes in the way obese patients metabolize carbohydrates during depression. These changes coincide with periods of greatest weight gain.[12] Dr. Jean Mayer colorfully characterizes depression-motivated overeating as "from gloom to gluttony."

IS YOUR REDUCING REGIME ADEQUATE?

Make sure the diet you choose for slenderizing is complete in kinds and amounts of nutrients needed, or you may take an emotional slide down into depression that could torture you into overeating and then hating yourself for doing it.

As several studies have shown, prisoner-of-war diets, notoriously deficient in nutrients, transformed many normal men into anxious, morbid, and depressed individuals. Similarly, many low-calorie diets can cause depression, fatigue, irritability, and lack of interest in sex—any one of which can compound already existing emotional stress and encourage compensatory overeating.

Members of the vitamin B family often are neglected in low-calorie diets, bringing on apathy, anxiety, restlessness, depression, irritability, forgetfulness, hair-trigger temper, nervousness and, among other symptoms, inability to sleep.

A deficiency of vitamin B-1 has been found to intensify or magnify already existing emotional problems. By its very nature, a diet high in refined carbohydrates may cause a deficiency of vitamins B-1, B-2, and B-6, required for making these very carbohydrates available to the body and mind. For example, sugarcane contains the B vitamins necessary for the assimilation of its sugar. However, refined sugar has been stripped of these essential vitamin helpers. Therefore, these B vitamins must be ingested in the foods or as supplements in order for the refined sugar to be assimilated. Likewise, refined flour, junk foods, and alcohol require similar assistance. A deficiency of B vitamins is the main reason alcoholics often are nervous, tremulous, irritable, and anxious, and eventually suffer hallucinations and even delirium tremens.

If the slenderizing diet you try to follow month after month is low in niacin, count on Blue Mondays seven days of the week, depression, feelings of hurt, abuse, or irritability.

If your low-calorie, slimming diet is deficient in pantothenic acid, expect a swarm of negative emotions: depression, irritability, hot temper, anti-sociability, quarrelsomeness, and generally delicate emotional balance—all of which contribute to biochemical stress and a desire, if not a lust, to overeat.

If you are on an unsupplemented, low-calorie reducing diet and on the Pill, too, bank on a host of negative emotions, due to a deficiency of vitamin B-6. Several studies reveal that the hormones in oral contraceptive pills deplete the body of this vitamin and invite mild to severe depression. I recommend that my patients who take the Pill ingest 50 mg of vitamin B-6 even on a normal diet.

Vitamin B-6 is a necessity for metabolizing tryptophan, an essential amino acid. Deficiency of either of these food elements may cause depression. Primary food sources of tryptophan are nuts, soybeans, tuna, and turkey, particularly the white meat.

Likewise, a deficiency of folic acid (or folate), another B family member, can contribute to depression, too. Scientists at McGill University in Montreal examined levels of blood folate in three types of patients—the depressed, the psychiatrically ill, and the medically ill. Blood folic acid levels were lower in the depressed than in the psychiatrically and medically ill patients.

In a published paper describing the study, A. Missagh Ghaderian, M.D., of McGill's department of psychiatry, concluded that "folic acid deficiency depression may exist."[13]

I have found that hypoglycemia can initiate and intensify depression, anxiety, confusion, antisocial behavior, crying jags, and various phobias.

So can hypothyroidism, as I have observed on numerous occasions. Whatever the origin of depression, anxiety, and related emotions, they are enemies to any weight-loss program in that they usually push you into overeating. This is especially true if you are already overweight and on the way to obesity and experiencing negative emotions that contribute to adding unwanted poundage.

You can be your own best friend if you become aware of and eliminate high-calorie emotions along with high-calorie foods.

10 | Why You Should Use Fat as a Motivating Force

So far Dr. Langer's weight loss program has dealt mainly with medical disorders that cause overweight and how difficult it is to lose poundage unless you cope with them first.

Now we shift gears into motivation, the next key phase to consider. If fat is your greatest liability, you can turn it into your greatest asset, a powerful, driving force. And this chapter will show you the medical reasons why you should.

Scare stories have circulated for decades about the serious physical consequences of obesity and, in many instances, even moderate overweight.

Pros and cons on this subject have been swatted back and forth like the shuttlecock in a badminton game. What's the truth on this subject?

Latest research indicates that the scare stories have not been scary enough.

However, a serious exception to the blubbery-fat generalization that obesity is associated with premature death from cardiovascular disease should be dealt with first.

The major risk of cardiovascular complication is within a subgroup of the obese, those who feature abdominal fat, as opposed to those who have a different distribution of adiposity.

Several epidemiological studies indicate that fat men and women with abdominal obesity are most prone to develop ischemic heart disease (medical jargon for the condition of insufficient blood supply to the Great Pump), stroke, and dying, regardless of the total degree of obesity.

A review study in the *Annals of Clinical Research* warns that even limited abdominal obesity should be treated along with other medical conditions contributing to obesity. So don't try to take refuge in the fact that your paunch may not be super large![1]

Here's how to determine whether or not you are obese in a health-hazardous way. If a tape measure shows that the circumference of your waist exceeds that of your hips, beware! Then work to reduce it.

Morbid obesity rockets a person into a higher risk category than does mere obesity. But, believe me, no obesity is really *mere*. Death rates of the morbidly obese are eleven times higher than those of the non-obese, reveals a study involving men only.[2] However, the same journal article offers the seeming contradiction that ''many obese patients are in apparent good health for years.''

THE PERIL OF BELLY FAT

So far as the risk factor of belly fat is concerned, a 13-year study of 722 54-year-old men in Gothenburg, Sweden, disclosed that other measures of obesity—the body mass index (BMI), the sum of three skinfold thickness—were incidental to significant waist-to-hip circumference comparison relative to the occurrence of stroke and ischemic heart disease.[3]

Results of the study were summed up in these words: ''. . . In middle-aged men, the distribution of fat deposits may be a better predictor of cardiovascular disease and death than the degree of adiposity.''

Another study, this one involving 5,506 test subjects ages 30 to 59, offers strong evidence of increased risk of hypertension (high blood pressure) as well in persons with belly fat.[4]

Still other investigations reveal that generalized obesity and hypertension frequently coexist. These disorders impose a heavy burden on the heart, particularly stressing the heart's left ventricle. Common to obesity and hypertension are congestive heart failure, coronary heart disease, and sudden death. However, weight loss reduced the degree of blood pressure and cardiac output.[5]

If you are obese, weight reduction diminishes the double load on the heart and should be your major objective for the prevention and treatment of heart disease.

Obesity hypertension is a problem not only for adults but often for their children, as shown by a case control study in Sweden. A review of 121 hypertensives, compared with 138 non-hypertensive controls, showed that parental obesity combined with hypertension proved to be a stronger risk indicator of hypertension in children than just parental hypertension.[6]

DURATION OF OBESITY: A CRITICAL MATTER

Added to obesity and distribution of fat as a health hazard is the duration of obesity, as indicated by one research project. The latter factor is important in causing thickening of the heart's left ventrical wall and determining the heart's dimension, stroke volume, and output. These features in thirty-five obese patients were compared with those in non-obese controls.[7]

One group of super-heavyweights had been obese for less than fifteen years. The second group had been obese for more than fifteen years. Both groups were of approximately the same weight and had fat cells of almost the same size. Both groups showed ventrical enlargement and alterations in heart performance compared with non-obese controls. However, those who had been obese longer showed significantly greater thickening of the heart's left ventrical wall and added ventricular dimension, an indication that duration of excess body weight compounds the harm done by obesity.

A related study demonstrated that substantial weight loss can reverse left ventricular dysfunction to some degree in morbidly obese patients.[8]

Research by the National Heart Foundation of Australia involving 5,550 male and female subjects aged 24 to 64 years revealed that obesity in terms of body-mass index was significantly and independently associated with blood pressure levels in both sexes. A maximum of 30 percent of hypertension could be attributed to overweight.[9]

OVERWEIGHT AND HIGH BLOOD PRESSURE

It is noteworthy that 60 percent of the hypertension in men under 45 years of age was related to overweight. Overweight hypertensives given medication to reduce blood pressure were less likely to achieve normal blood pressure than non-overweights, according to the authors of this study.

Not every obese or overweight person develops high blood pressure, of course, but there is a close association between these conditions and hypertension in all age groups, states a review article in *Biomedical Pharmacotherapy*.[10]

In addition to over-nutrition and intake of too much sodium, contributors to the development of hypertension in obesity are hyperinsulinemia and insulin-induced sodium retention.

The writers of this paper recommend lower food intake and increased physical activity for reduction of hypertension in the obese. As insulin levels decline on this regime, sodium absorption in the kidneys may also decrease.

Weight loss does not lower blood pressure in all cases, however. When this does occur, it usually decreases before weight reduction reaches the normal level. Reducing sodium intake does not appear to explain why weight loss lowers blood pressure.

Since hypertension is not the only cardiovascular risk factor in the obese, glucose intolerance and high level of blood fats—both of which contribute to atherosclerosis—should also be considered. Normalizing of weight by diet and increased exercise are the most crucial steps in therapy.

LOSE WEIGHT, LOSE HYPERTENSION

Significant lowering of blood pressure can also be achieved through weight loss by those who are merely overweight, not just the obese. This was revealed in an experiment with young test subjects that compared success in controlling hypertension by weight reduction or by taking an anti-hypertensive, metoprolol.[11]

All 56 patients had diastolic blood pressure of 90 to 109 mm Hg. Placebo controls were also used. After 21 weeks, those trying to reduce lost an average of 7.4 kg (roughly 16 pounds). Their systolic pressure dropped markedly more than that of the placebo group: 13 mm Hg, contrasted with seven mm Hg, but not significantly different from the metoprolol group: 10 mm Hg.

However, the weight loss group's drop in diastolic pressure was 10 mm Hg, appreciably greater than that of the metoprolol takers, 6 mm Hg, and that of the placebo group: 3 mm Hg. Further, 50 percent of the weight-reduction group's diastolic reading had gone below 90 mm Hg—to normal levels.

So far as blood fats are concerned, the metoprolol patients showed a decrease in high-density lipoproteins (HDL), the protective Good Guy cholesterol, and an increase in the ratio of total cholesterol to HDL. Not so with the weight-reduction patients. Their cholesterol decreased and so did the ratio of total cholesterol to HDL. The weight-reduction group had higher grades in reducing blood pressure without the adverse effects on blood fats common to those on the anti-hypertensive drug.

Raising of the HDL-cholesterol level is usually desirable insurance against diseases of arteries and heart. An experiment with forty obese female subjects revealed that losing weight frequently brings on HDL-cholesterol elevation.[12]

Even more effective in increasing HDL cholesterol is the combination of weight loss and exercise, as indicated by an experiment with twenty-one obese sedentary men.[13]

OBESITY: INVITATION TO ILLNESS

Over and above cardiovascular disorders, obesity—even overweight—appears to invite a host of diseases: cancer, diabetes, respiratory ailments, gallstones, and other medical conditions.

A twelve-year investigation by the American Cancer Society

showed that obesity increases the risk of many types of cancer: breast, colon, gallbladder, kidney, stomach, and uterus. Neither sex is spared.[14]

Men 40 percent overweight are 33 percent more prone to develop cancer than those of normal weight. Women 40 percent or more overweight are at even greater risk of developing cancer than those of normal weight: 55 percent greater. Several animal studies have demonstrated similar findings.

In a breast cancer screening for fifty-year-old-plus women with determination of estrogen-receptor (ER) status of cancers, cancer was favored by obesity and relatively inhibited by leanness. Leanness in post-menopausal women appears to encourage ER-negative cells in cancers.[15]

Researchers in this study state that obesity does not seem to initiate breast cancer, but it does encourage the spread of existing cancer. Tumors that are present appear to grow if they receive stimulus to which they are sensitive. Obesity appears to be a stimulus, rather than an initiator.

A little-known contributor to fatal prostate cancer is obesity, indicate findings of a 20-year study of 6,763 white, male, Seventh Day Adventists. Overweight males had a significantly higher amount of prostate cancer than males of normal weight.[16]

MISHANDLING CARBOHYDRATES

As with cancer, diabetes mellitus appears to be aided and abetted by obesity. There is an amazing similarity in how the body handles carbohydrates in diabetes and in obesity, states Dr. W. John Butterfield, professor of medicine at Guys Hospital in London.[17] Comparative cell uptake of glucose was tested in three groups of patients: juvenile diabetics, maturity-onset diabetics, and normal control test subjects. Juvenile diabetics could not absorb sugar (glucose) in their cells, evidence that they suffered a deficit of internally secreted insulin.

Uptake of glucose by older diabetics and grossly overweight normal subjects was almost identical. Lean control subjects took up more sugar than plump individuals.

Butterfield observed that obese patients handled carbohydrates similarly to diabetics. With the increase and duration of obesity, less insulin is delivered to insulin-responsive muscles. In order for glucose to make it through cell walls, where it can be used for energy, it must be escorted through by insulin with an assist from the trace mineral chromium, which acts as a catalyst.

With less glucose uptake in obesity, the pancreas is forced to form more insulin. As obesity increases, the pancreas can't always produce enough insulin to meet demand. This results in hyperglycemia. Butterfield indicates that reversible obesity diabetes is actually a breakdown of the body's insulin-glucose economy. There is a battle between the fat and muscle for the available insulin. The fat wins, and this leads to another unwanted result: carbohydrates are changed into more fat.

In a multi-year, follow-up study of 288 subjects with borderline glucose tolerance, large maximum-body-weight index, and a diminished insulin response to glucose load proved significant risk factors in this condition worsening and becoming diabetes.[18]

Diabetes occurred almost exclusively in the low-insulin responders among 253 non-obese or mildly obese test subjects. Some of 35 grossly obese test subjects—normal to high insulin responders—developed diabetes. The researchers concluded that the majority of cases of non-insulin-dependent diabetes mellitus resulted from low insulin secretion, with an added precipitating factor of obesity. In a number of test subjects with high insulin responses, diabetes occurred along with gross obesity.

UPPER BODY FAT CONTRIBUTES TO DIABETES

Another study reveals a startling discovery: that, as in obesity-related cardiovascular disorders, fat concentrated in one specific area is more important in pushing individuals over the line into diabetes than generally distributed adiposity.[19]

Prominent fat in the upper part of the body is the chief factor that contributes to developing diabetes. There is a special name for this configuration of fat: diabetogenic and atherogenic obesity.

The researchers indicate that this type of obesity progresses in five stages of initial obesity without diabetes to insulin-dependent diabetes. The biochemical mechanism that starts this progression is still not known. Non-insulin-dependent diabetes has its onset in adult years—particularly accompanying obesity in women more than in men. I have seen this tendency in my practice and in several studies. One that appeared in the *American Journal of Clinical Nutrition* accents this point and the fact that diabetes was repeated more often as obesity increased, especially at advanced ages.[20]

Obesity is among the "Big Three" major environmental factors influencing the development of non-insulin-dependent diabetes mellitus in those with the genes for it. The others are excessive caloric intake (leading to obesity) and physical inactivity. Still other contributors are various forms of stress, hormonal imbalance, drugs, toxins, and the aging process, as shown in a study reported in the *American Journal of Medicine*.[21]

The researchers recommend that treatment or prevention of non-insulin dependent diabetes mellitus be aimed at eliminating environmental factors contributing to insulin-resistance—particularly obesity and those that increase insulin sensitivity.

PREGNANCY COMPLICATED BY OBESITY

Obesity's influence on one's physical condition covers the full spectrum of medical ailments, including obstetrics. Are there special risks to mother and her infant in moderate obesity?

Definitely!

Two researchers conducted a partially computerized search of literature in this special area, papers covering controlled studies of 10,440 cases over a 22-year period.[22]

Thirty-seven complications were found to be significantly more prevalent in the obese subjects than in lean controls. However, because data were frequently conflicting, the searchers listed only solidly documented complications of pregnancy: preeclampsia—and separate elements of this disorder—diabetes mellitus, varicose veins, and the necessity for caesarian section.

One possible surprise is the fact that significantly higher birth weight of infants did not cause an increase of labor complications.

OBESITY AND GALLBLADDER TROUBLES

Notorious among disorders common to the obese of both sexes is gallbladder trouble, including gallstones. Grossly obese patients are prime candidates for developing cholesterol gallstones, as researchers discovered by collecting gallbladder bile at surgery from massively obese patients. Bile was significantly more saturated with cholesterol than bile from non-obese patients matched for age, sex, and gallstone status.[23]

Even treatment of gallstones during a five-week therapy of chenodeoxycholic acid was not as effective in reducing cholesterol saturation in bile of the massively obese patients.

The bile of four out of ten obese patients remained supersaturated, compared with one out of ten non-obese subjects.

The study concludes that cholesterol saturation of bile is raised in gross obesity and the ability to respond to treatment with chenodeoxycholic acid is lessened—which would explain why obese patients respond poorly to the dissolving of gallstones with bile acid.

BREATHING RESTRICTED

As with gallbladder problems, obesity even influences something as basic as breathing. Difficulty in breathing experienced by many of the obese is caused by fat restricting chest expansion and, therefore, intake of air, as illustrated by experiments described in the publication *Respiration*.[24]

The researchers conclude that this is the main reason for a change in breathing. The condition worsens with passing time and influences air capacity, flow, and discharge of carbon dioxide.

Some of the major complications associated with obesity are revealed in a study of twelve massively obese patients: 5

women and 7 men, ages 25 to 59 years and weighing from 312 to more than 500 pounds, an average of 381 pounds.[25]

The study found hypertension (experienced by seven patients), herpomania or sleep apnea (four patients), diabetes mellitus (two patients), and coronary artery disease (one patient). Five patients died suddenly from undeterminable causes, two from right-sided congestive heart failure, one from acute myocardial infarction, one from aortic dissection, one from intracerebral hemorrhage, one from a drug overdose, and another following an ileal bypass.

Every patient showed increased heart weight. The left ventricular heart cavity was dilated in eleven patients, and the right ventricular cavity in all twelve.

Despite warnings from medical doctors of obesity's serious consequences—even of moderate overweight, depending upon location of fat—many patients shrug them off.

Unfortunately, the threat of ill health and earlier death than necessary motivates patients far less than we wish.

The typical attitude is reflected in results of a survey published in the *Journal of the American Dietetic Association.* Four hundred female college students were asked, among other things, to state their strongest motive for losing weight. Most of them responded, ''Improved appearance!''[26]

The next chapter will penetrate a little deeper into how you can motivate yourself to lose.

11 | How to Change Won't Power to Will Power

Goal orientation is just as important in weight loss as in career.

Be specific about your goal, such as, "I want to lose forty pounds in ten months."

Also be realistic about your goal and the time required to reach it. (You've already been burned by those alluring ads that promise you a twenty-pound weight loss overnight!) If you're not realistic, discouragement will soon douse your motivational fire.

Remember, you put on that padding on the installment plan, and you're going to have to take it off by the installment plan— in small installments, too.

Motivation is not quite enough. It must be *sustained motivation.*

That's the nub of the problem. You say to yourself, "I've been here before. Sustained motivation sounds good on paper, but I can't accomplish it."

Yes, you can!

THE DAVIS SYSTEM OF MOTIVATION

In order to show you how, I must use the method of a successful man in executive placement. Lee Andre Davis, president of Davis Executives in Westlake Village in southern California, has a special way to motivate clients, some of whom he places in six-figure salary positions.

But let's start at the beginning. Losing a job is something like failing to lose weight. It can be a devastating experience. With the loss of a job often come discouragement, diminished self-esteem, and difficulty in motivating yourself to get back into the executive marketplace.

Lee Davis insists that all new applicants fill out a lengthy questionnaire in detail, starting with defining clear-cut career goals and then listing major contributions they have made to companies with which they have been affiliated. Lee also asks for details about special awards, recognition, and publicity they've received for contributions to the community and/or the world.

Some devastated, unemployed executives rebel at the brain-cudgeling and soul-searching this takes, saying, "I came here for a new position, not to spend the rest of my life filling out a questionnaire."

It is an *either/or* situation with Davis. Those who won't fill out the questionnaire are out the door because the questionnaire has a special purpose beyond the obvious one. Answered conscientiously and in depth, it reminds the applicant of the positive contributions he or she has made and the achievements scored. It rebuilds self-esteem and recharges flagging motivation.

Davis also holds monthly meetings of applicants and spouses to show how wives and husbands can keep a positive, supportive atmosphere at home—excellent for backing a weight-loss program, too.

Like executives applying at Davis Executives, you have experienced one or more discouraging setbacks in your weight-loss programs, sometimes even regaining more poundage than you had lost. As you look back and shudder, you realize that all you have to show for your hard efforts is a greater bank balance of fat.

THE POWER OF POSITIVISM

You need something positive to get yourself moving again. So what that your track record looks bad! Let me tell you how the Davis system worked for one of my heavy-weight patients.

Erika stood about five-foot-five in stocking feet and weighed 180 pounds. Every dress in her wardrobe felt like a straitjacket. It was a major production for her to pull, tug, and struggle into her girdle. She was exhausted when she woke up in the morning from hauling around her excess fat the day before. Due to her full figure, Erika had another problem. The shoulder straps of her bra cut into her flesh. Misery seemed to have been invented just for her.

"I can never stay on a weight-loss program long enough to do any good," she had sighed.

I had Erika fill out several pages of paper about accomplishments and awards she had received, particularly those scored over a considerable time span.

It turned out that in junior high school, Erika had created a miniature colonial village, stockade, inner buildings, trees, and even people. Several months of after-school work had paid off. She had won first prize in the school exhibit. Her creation was borrowed by the local chamber of commerce and, later, by a large manufacturing firm for exhibition.

Then, by her own admission, Erika, not too graceful on skis, had put in months of arduous hours on the snow-covered hills near her home in the north Midwest. Over the years, she had mastered ski-jumping, even winning several competitions in college.

Recalling her accomplishments and the acclaim she had won through goal orientation and sustained motivation gave her new hope. This time she established a weight-loss goal: to be able to fit into a black bikini by losing fifty-five pounds in one year.

The Mega Weight Loss Diet, offered in Chapter 21, fed rather than starved Erika. That and a regular exercise program, thirty minutes of brisk walking, slowly whittled off the fat. She sustained her motivation by reminding herself of previous successes. What she had done before, she could do again. And she did. Within a year, Erika fitted neatly into that black bikini. Now she also has new energy, more zest for living, and higher self-esteem.

There are other Erikas in my case files, too, as well as Johns and Roys who searched and found the motivations they could sustain. And they lost the desired amount of weight.

DO YOU HAVE A BLACK BIKINI?

Turning won't power into willpower is not always easy, but it's always possible if you use the Davis system and if you take one day at a time. Everybody has his or her equivalent of Erika's black bikini. Before we get into some equivalents, let me tell you how another patient of mine multiplied the influence of the black bikini to supermotivate herself. She taped it to the refrigerator door!

One of my male patients—tired of being blubbery fat and ever-exhausted from carrying around his excess weight—had been a slim, trim, browned lifeguard twelve years earlier.

"I don't dare visit the beach anymore," he complained. "I'm afraid I'll be harpooned."

Chuck had found a pair of swim trunks he had worn while a lifeguard and decided to make fitting into them his goal.

It looked hopeless to me, like the grapes that tantalized Tantalus, but at least he had a clear-cut goal. To his credit, Chuck shaped every day's thoughts and activities to the objective of fitting into those trunks—first walking, then jogging for 25 minutes daily, and swimming in his pool five times a week. He followed his 1,500-calorie diet religiously.

Chuck lost twenty pounds in the first two months.

"Now that I'm beginning to look human again, I'm encouraged to go on," he told me.

In the next two months, he dropped fifteen more pounds. Then he was transferred to the company's plant in the Southeast.

That was the last I saw of him. However, six months later, I received an envelope in the mail postmarked Atlanta. There was a brief note from Chuck and a large color photo of him in swim trunks.

No, he hadn't lost enough poundage to fit into his old swimming trunks, but he hadn't lost his sense of humor. The note read: "Old Chinese proverb: a picture tells more than a thousand words. I wish I could say I'm wearing my old swim trunks, but I can't. However, I have rid myself of 75 pounds—as you can see—and feel fantastic. I've taped my old swim trunks to the refrigerator door. Great motivation. I may never fit into the oldies, but I fit into these new ones pretty well. Thanks for your help, doctor!''

TRY THESE MOTIVATIONS FOR SIZE

Maybe the black bikini or the old swim trunks aren't for you. Okay, here are some other motivations you can dramatize to sustain your drive to lower weight:

1. Just looking slender and more shapely for Mr. Right or for Ms. Right;

2. Regaining a feeling of mastery over your appetite and an overfat body that has taken you over;

3. Overcoming depressing symptoms of ill health and feeling bouncy, optimistic, and vigorous again;

4. Getting into shape for a long-sought, elusive job promotion (overweight sometimes blocks career advancement);

5. Recapturing the feeling of youth that slenderness often brings;

6. Having more energy for work, play, accomplishment, and well-being.

If these motivations which have helped so many of my patients are not right for you, search your heart and find power-house motivations that *will* work for you.

Then get moving toward your goal. It won't come to you. Start today. If you do, you'll be one day closer to realization than if you start tomorrow.

Excuses and rationalizations lead to putting off what you should be taking off. Procrastination is not only ''the thief of time,'' it is the thief of motivation, realization, self-esteem, and good health.

EXCUSES, EXCUSES, EXCUSES!

Don't hide behind the following pet excuses to defer your slenderizing regime:

1. "My birthday party is set for this weekend, so I'll start dieting next Monday."

(Yeah, and after your birthday will come your nephew Jason's wedding, "All you can eat" night at your nearby restaurant, and then that ten-day cruise through the Panama Canal with loads of tempting foods and gooey desserts a mile high with whipped cream. Start on your low-calorie diet right now. Then you can lose a little before your birthday. If weight loss is really important, skip Jason's wedding and send him and his bride a nice gift. Also, defer the cruise for a while—say, a lifetime.)

2. "I'm not feeling well enough to reduce my calories now."

(How much better will you feel three months from now with ten more pounds of gut and butt?)

3. "I'm too exhausted to go without foods I need and to start exercising now."

(Are you going to feel less tired six months and fifteen pounds later?)

4. "People I lunch with near the office will think I'm a spoilsport if I don't join them in a martini and eat heartily and have a rich dessert with them."

(Hey, it's your life as well as your figure that raises the bathtub water. You owe yourself something, too. As for the dessert and your friends, order a fresh fruit cup without whipped cream, and let 'em eat cake!)

5. "Waiters at my favorite restaurants will feel hurt if I don't eat everything on my plate!"

(Hurt, schmurt! Be a pleasant guest. Eat only what you need, and leave a generous tip.)

6. "I've tried all the weight-loss plans and none of them works for me."

(You haven't tested the Mega Weight Loss Diet, so how do you know?)

   7. "There's no use even attempting to motivate myself. My problem is in my glands."

(That's where the problem is, all right—in your salivary glands!)

   8. "I'll just keep waiting until they come up with some miracle pill."

(Forget it. If you have read the ads for the last few decades, you should know that there have been miracle pills and regimes ever since human beings began preying on other human beings. These pills and systems aren't quite miraculous enough. Delay your slenderizing program as you continue your present eating and exercising habits, and the situation can only get worse.)

THE HARD WAY IS THE EASIEST WAY

Let's be realistic.

You didn't become overweight overnight. You did it by degrees. Then all those little degrees began to add up. All of a sudden (it seemed) you were 20, 30, 40 or 100 percent more of a person than you were before.

You became what you are today by certain eating habits and certain non-exercising habits. It was the line of least resistance that now compels you to follow the line of most resistance—that is, if you are serious about wanting to lose weight.

Forget easy ways. Start out the hard way. Build new eating and exercising regimes. Hang in there with them minute-to-minute, hour-to-hour, day-to day, month-to-month, and soon a new habit system will have been formed—a habit system that will help you lose weight, slowly and surely, and keep it off.

Until now, your habits have been working against you. Now you can make them work for you. Many of my patients have done what I have suggested here. You can, too.

12 | New Behavior, New Figure

A threadbare cliché holds that "all the world loves a fat person."

Not so. The fat person often doesn't even like himself or herself. Neither does the company carrying his or her life insurance. And, speaking of insurance, obesity or even 20 percent overweight almost guarantees the person shorter life expectancy.

You will like yourself more if there's less of you. This chapter will show you why you may tend to overeat, and how to change your behavior patterns so that you can reduce temptation and be in command of your diet.

In my study of more than 1,200 articles on weight reduction in the world's medical journals, I found almost unanimous agreement that a single-phase approach to weight loss—diet, exercise, *or* behavior modification only—is doomed to failure.

Team up the three major approaches—diet, exercise, and behavior modification—and you can score with significant and permanent weight loss.

Let's look at behavior modification first. A successful four-year study of a combined behavioral modification program for long-term treatment of obesity reported in the *British Medical Journal* concludes:

". . . Combined behavioral modification used on a program for reducing weight may result in a substantial loss of weight for several years for severely obese subjects."

In my preventive medical practice, this is my experience, too. Basic behavioral modification is the name of the game. Life-style patterns that helped bring on your overweight in the first place must be modified.

HOW TO CHANGE HABIT PATTERNS

Before getting into the *how* of behavior modification, let me give you a sample of changes in habit patterns used with phenomenal success by Willem H. Khoe, M.D., Ph.D., of Las Vegas, Nevada. Many of my overweight patients have become good losers from it. The thanks I get should rightfully go to Dr. Khoe. Here in his own words is a guide for behavior modification:

1. "If you feel the urge to snack between meals and you know you shouldn't, go brush your teeth!"
(Dr. Khoe's patients have the most dazzling white smiles in Las Vegas.)

2. "Keep your scale in the kitchen—not in the bathroom—and weigh yourself often. The scale can reinforce your will and keep you from snacking.

3. "Buy a kitchen timer. Set it for ten minutes. Whenever it's mealtime and you feel like eating, take that ten-minute pause to think whether you really *want* to eat or not.

4. "When you are tempted to snack excessively, take a relaxing bath, a nap, or a walk.

(A brisk walk will take off some of the calories that a snack would have put on.)

5. "During meals, set the timer for 20 minutes. Always stretch out mealtime for at least that long. Studies show that it takes about 20 minutes for the brain to receive the message that the stomach is full. Setting a timer will help you cue into your body's sense of hunger.

(Excellent advice. Several studies show that the obese and significantly overweight eat fast, finishing their meals faster than the normal-weight persons.)

6. "Jot down in a notebook everything you eat, how you feel when you eat, and the persons you are with. At the end of the day, you can readily associate the triggering incidents, feelings, and individuals who may be leading you into overeating. Be forewarned and prepared.

7. "Eat in one established place at home. In other words, don't eat in the living room while watching TV, or in the den while reading or in the kitchen while talking on the phone. Absent-minded eating leads to overeating.

8. "Make eating a pleasure. Get a colorful place setting, plates and silverware. Turn on the music and put freshly cut flowers on the table. Light the candles. Many dieters have negative feelings about their desire to eat. However, it is important to dissipate those feelings. The more you enjoy what you eat, the more in control of the diet you will feel. The next result is eating less," Dr. Khoe concludes.

WHY YOU'RE TEMPTED TO OVEREAT

Over and above the Khoe ground rules, how can you design a behavioral modification program to discourage overeating? By basing it on two well-established findings:

1. Heavyweights, more than normal weights, are influenced by food cues to eat.

2. They are also more influenced by the pleasurable taste of food to overeat.

Psychologists have found that when food was made more visible by highlights or by being wrapped in transparent paper, the obese were far more motivated to eat than normal weights.[1]

In an experiment, obese and normal-weight test subjects were brought into a room by psychologist R. E. Nisbett on the pretext of participating in a study of psychological response. They were briefed, then led into a second room to respond to questionnaires and also invited to have a bottle of soft drink.[2]

At their desk, they found either one or three sandwiches that they were invited to eat, since they had missed lunch to take part in the study. They were also informed that there were more sandwiches in the refrigerator and that they could eat as many as they wished.

Left alone but still observed without their knowledge, the heavyweights ate more sandwiches than the slender individuals —2.32 to 1.88 average when three sandwiches were available. On the other hand, when one sandwich was in sight, the over-weight persons averaged only 1.48 sandwiches as opposed to 1.96 for the normal weights.

Another indication that obese persons are more motivated by seeing food is shown by a test of Drs. Stanley Schachter and Lucy Friedman.[3]

Forty obese and forty normal-weight individuals sat at pur-posely littered desks to fill out questionnaires, a task set up to divert them from the purpose of the experiment. On half of the desks was either a bag of unshelled or shelled almonds.

In both the normal and the obese groups, just one person out of twenty ate almonds that needed to be shelled. However, results were far different in the groups with the shelled, ready-to-eat almonds.

Eleven out of twenty of the normal-weight group ate the shelled nuts, as compared with nineteen out of twenty in the obese group. So what does this mean? That obese persons are more dependent on visual food cues and are more easily seduced into eating what's in sight.

BUT IT TASTES *SO GOOD!*

A second finding is that the obese are more turned on to overeat by the taste of a favored food than normal-weight sub-jects.

Two researchers compared the effect of taste upon degree of appetite in both weight categories with patients at the Nutrition Clinic of Saint Luke's Hospital in New York City.[4]

Prior to the experiment, obese test subjects had been eating some 3,500 calories daily as opposed to 2,200 calories consumed by the normal-weight group.

Then the obese participants' intake of food was cut to 2,400 calories for a week, followed by 1,200 calories in the next week. During the same two weeks, normal-weight patients were fed 2,400 calorie diets.

During the last week of the experiment, both groups were put on an almost tasteless, bland, liquid diet well-enriched with vitamins and minerals to ensure nutritional soundness. Normal-weight subjects continued to take in approximately the same diet. However, the obese subjects progressively reduced their intake until they were consuming an average of 500 calories daily.

Test results convinced the researchers that the degree of appetite in obese persons is more influenced by how satisfying the food tastes than it is in normal-weight individuals.

In another experiment to discover whether or not taste preference induces the obese to eat more, psychologists had obese and normal-weight persons skip a meal on the premise that they were part of an experiment to learn how hunger affects concentration.[5]

Upon completion of a questionnaire, one half of the group—equally divided between grossly overweight and normal-weight—were fed roast beef and Swiss cheese sandwiches. The other half received no food.

Without test subjects realizing it, they were then introduced to the heart of the experiment. They were offered as much ice cream as they wished from two sources: (1) supposedly a new flavor called *bitter vanilla*, regular vanilla treated with 2.5 grams of quinine sulphate per quart, and (2) regular sweet vanilla. Invariably, obese test participants out-ate normal-weight subjects per gram of the ice cream that appealed to their taste, regardless of whether they had eaten sandwiches earlier.

Although the facts of the study made a convincing point, researcher R. E. Nisbett puzzled over a troubling question: Were test results due to the individuals being overweight or were they a cause of overweight?

So he checked on the amounts of ice cream (measured in grams) consumed by normal-weight subjects who, over a lifetime, had had bouts with overweight. Invariably, this category of person ate markedly more of the flavorful ice cream and much less of the "bitter vanilla."

Similar experiments have been done with tasty and "doctored" cake, and with regular vanilla milk shakes and doctored vanilla milk shakes, with the same results.[6]

Additional proof that heavyweights are more motivated by external cues to overeat resulted from an experiment in which psychologists manipulated test participants by moving clocks ahead to make them think it was dinner time.

Overweight persons ate nearly twice as much food when they thought it was 6:15 p.m. as when the clock showed 5:20 p.m. Much more evidence demonstrates that the eating of overweight persons is triggered mainly by outside cues—time of day, appearance, taste and smell of foods, as well as the sight of others eating. At the other pole are normal-weight individuals who are moved to eat mainly by internal cues—stomach contractions and low blood sugar.

Still another study proves the same point: that heavyweights are inclined to follow where their taste buds lead. Columbia University undergraduates suffer a penalty of $15 for cancelling meal contracts at institutional cafeterias in favor of more appealing off-campus restaurants. It was found that 86.5 percent of fat undergraduates cancelled their meal contracts, compared to 57.1 percent of normal-weight students.[7]

Again, taste proved to be a more dominant force among the heavyweights than among the normal weights. Two facts have been established by these studies: (1) that food cues stimulate the obese more than the non-obese; and that (2) taste induces the obese to eat greater quantities of favored foods than it does for normal-weight persons.

KEEP FOOD FROM TURNING YOU ON

What bearing do these findings have on the overweight? External cues and appealing taste stimulate their appetites and induce them to overeat. However, these factors can be used in reverse as the foundation for a behavioral modification plan: avoiding food cues and minimizing use of favorite foods.

The key to turning off food cues that turn you on is never to let them get to you. Avoiding them is far easier than fighting them.

Keep tempting foods out of the house. One of my formerly obese patients used to say: "If there are chocolates in the house, I eat the whole box to get rid of the temptation."

In the process of avoiding food cues and the foods themselves, the best bet is to make tempting areas of your supermarket off limits. If you, an overeater, enter these forbidden zones, you are vulnerable. The food has you where it wants you.

Companies that process and package foods—as well as their Madison Avenue agents—are masters of every psychological ploy to prey on your weaknesses. Displays of creamy cakes, chocolate-nuggeted cookies, colorful soft drinks, and golden, crisp, crunchy chips and snacks seem to find every chink in your armor.

When I told a rather well-padded patient that the contest between her and the food processors was subtle seduction, she smiled and corrected me:

"So far as I'm concerned, it's rape."

All right. Avoidance is the first preventive measure. What more?

Time your shopping correctly. Shop for food just after having eaten. A full stomach is your second line of defense. Satiation takes the edge off temptation when faced with hard-to-resist foods. Several studies indicate that the best time to shop is after dinner.

After-dinner shoppers bought 19.7 percent less food than before-dinner shoppers. When the shopping time of both test subject groups was reversed on another day, the after-dinner shoppers bought 15.7 percent less than the other group.

CREATE A MINI OBSTACLE COURSE

Here's a cardinal rule. Never do spontaneous shopping for food. Fight your temptation at home by scribbling a list of diet-acceptable foods that you plan to buy. Do not budge from this shopping list.

Another buttress against impulsive, diet-wrecking purchasing is to bring along only enough money to pay for foods on the list.

Despite your best intentions, sometimes you must buy foods for other members of the family, for company, or simply because the store is too far away to make repeated trips.

Then, your best move is to put them out of sight in the deepest recess of the cupboard or the refrigerator. You can't very well build an obstacle course between yourself and the foods, and it isn't practical to gird your refrigerator with a strong link chain and padlock it.

However, you don't have to go to extremes. Even slight impediments will help you resist. If it is necessary to buy your nemesis foods, buy them in a form that requires preparation before use: the mixing of ingredients, or cooking and baking.

As another example, let's say you want to eat a slice of bread and are trying to resist making it two. Develop the habit of toasting it. Preparing more than one slice will lead to eating more. Make it an inflexible rule to put away the rest of the loaf prior to eating. Then sit at a table in the dining room. The farther away from the additional bread, the better. Now, in order to eat more toast, you have to follow a lengthy procedure: going to the refrigerator for a second slice, placing it in the toaster, putting the rest of the bread back in the refrigerator, returning to the table, sitting down and eating.

The fact that it's too much like work to eat a second slice is discouraging, interrupting what would have been an automatic eating of that additional slice—and, at the same time, giving you various stages in the procedure at which you can say, "Do I really need that second slice?"

Obstacles are important. Remember the resistance to eating the unshelled almonds mentioned earlier? Plan your day's eating. Set a daily goal: a specific number of calories, permitting only snacks within that quota, and avoiding people and situations that tempt overeating.

EFFECTIVE DEVICES

Don't fail to tell people you are on a diet. This will accomplish two important objectives: usually friends and co-workers will cooperate by not tempting you and may even reinforce your intentions and efforts; making a public commitment to your goal will act as a social control over your eating, too.

Either at home or out, serve yourself smaller helpings. At home you can use smaller plates, which will make you take smaller quantities. Never leave the serving platter in front of you. This only encourages multiple helpings. If you can't resist dessert or don't want to offend your host or hostess, request a small helping.

As I said earlier, goal orientation is as important to melting away flab as it is in career success. Make it a point never to eat while watching TV, attending a sports event, or seeing a film in a theater. Instead, suck on a no-calorie mint or chew sugarless gum.

If you must snack at work or at home, do it with nutritious, low-calorie food: carrot sticks, celery, a slice of cheese, or a small apple. Challenge yourself by slowly lengthening the intervals between snacks, keeping score so that you can gain reinforcement by bettering your previous day's record.

And, speaking of reinforcement, when you've lost a few pounds, reward yourself with non-eating pleasures. Positive reinforcement is an important tool in behavioral modification. Everybody has certain pleasurable activities that he or she finds rewarding: playing golf, buying a stereo tape or a book, seeing a play.

LIST YOUR TEMPTATIONS

Some weight-control authorities recommend keeping detailed records on all foods eaten—where, when, with whom, and the caloric value of each item. These are important details to help you modify your habit patterns. However, such record keeping imposes such a burden that overweight patients soon abandon it.

A simpler way is to make a list of temptations that cause you to overeat—for instance, watching TV or having too many of your favorite foods on hand. Rather than keep detailed books, merely cut an hour or two off your TV time. This will spare you exposure to tempting food ads. (It is a good idea to leave the room during food commercials.) It will also give you less time to eat unconsciously while viewing.

In place of lost TV time, substitute pleasurable alternate activities: a walk in the park, a jog with a friend, a game of billiards, reading a book or a magazine.

Now about your favorite foods. Here's how to eat fewer of them. If ice cream is your nemesis, buy a flavor that has little appeal to you. This will lessen your intake and may well prevent you from going on an ice cream binge.

Remember what you read in the chapter *Lose Allergies and Weight*—particularly the fact that we tend to be addicted to and have food sensitivities or allergies to our favorites. By minimizing them or even eliminating them, if possible, you can speed your weight loss.

Don't forget about rotating your foods, not eating any one of them more than every fifth day. Although we have concentrated on food and eating in this chapter, behavior modification is by no means limited to this area.

For your weight-control program to succeed, you will also have to modify your behavior relative to physical activity, with an accent on increased exercise.

13 | Win the Losing Battle with Exercise

Behavior modification not only can help you eat less to lose weight, it can also help you exercise more for the same purpose.

Don't be discouraged about starting physical activity even if you've spent most of your days in an office chair, accumulating ballast and exercising only your imagination.

Thanks to the weight-loss program outlined in this book, you can blend easy-to-do, fat-melting exercise into your day without disturbing your usual routine.

However, you may be reluctant to exercise more—or at all—because of persistent, discouraging, and erroneous myths about exercise: (1) that physical activity contributes little to weight loss (probably promoted by the obese who find it easier to sit than to move or by writers of diet books); and (2) that added exercise only makes you eat more, so that its influence on weight loss is cancelled out.

Let's deal with Myth Number One first. If physical exercise has little influence on weight loss, answer these questions.

Why are geese and pigs penned in and overfed before going to market? Why are cattle taken off the open range, confined to close quarters in feedlots, and liberally fed before going to market?

The obvious answer is: to gain weight because they are sold by the pound.

In many instances—if not most—you gain weight by the same formula: too little exercise and too much food.

Why did the National Research Council make its Recommended Dietary Allowances (RDAs) vary according to amount of physical activity? Why did this organization set a 2,400-calorie diet for inactive men? Why 4,500 calories for very active men and up to 6,000 calories for heavy laborers (miners, lumberjacks, farmers, field soldiers, and athletes)?

The answers are self-evident.

Now let's deal with Myth Number Two. Those who pooh-pooh exercise for weight loss make statements such as: "It would take a half hour a day of vigorous jogging over twenty-one days to lose a pound."

This is a lot of work for a small benefit. They argue that by refusing a daily piece of pie (400 calories) for 24 days, you could bring about a weight loss of five pounds. Yes, if you can resist the temptation of the pie.

THE GWINUP SECRET OF EFFICIENT LOSING

Dr. Grant Gwinup, professor of metabolism and endocrinology at the University of California, Irvine, and author of more than fifty publications on weight control, says:

"Exercising is far more effective than dieting in getting rid of excess weight. Individuals who diet without exercising lose mainly water and some muscle.

"When you're not eating enough food, when you're relying *only* on dieting to lose weight, your body fights back. It lowers your metabolic rate. That's why your weight tends to plateau," says Dr. Gwinup. "However, if you exercise strenuously for 30 minutes or more daily, you will burn off fat and keep muscle. You may not even have to cut down on food."[1]

The anti-exercise argument that you will need to jog vigorously for twenty-one days to lose a pound doesn't take into account that aerobic exercise speeds up the body's metabolism.

"Fat is burned off at a much faster rate," Dr. Gwinup continues. "Remember that the fat-burning process goes on for several hours after a vigorous workout. This means that meals that are eaten within that period are metabolized faster."

If you are physically inactive, you invite fat to settle in your fat cells. Remember, glycogen is stored in the liver and tissues to be released in the form of glucose when your blood sugar goes too low. However, it needs a trigger. That trigger is adrenalin, released under emotional or physical stimulation. Glucagon, a pancreatic hormone, is secreted when you exercise and the liver has to replace burned-up glucose.

A few generations ago, human beings were far more physically active in making a living and struggling for survival. Today, rather than working hard while standing, most of us work sitting down, expending little physical energy.

In our forty hours or less of work each week, we release little adrenalin or glucagon, except while under stress. So our glycogen bank account is high, but the blood-sugar level starts to drop in mid-morning and mid-afternoon. Hunger begins to demand attention, although we have been relatively inactive physically. We differ from the ditch digger whose revved-up metabolism has used up his blood sugar and much or all of his stored glycogen. This leads to *honest* hunger.

The desk worker's hunger is of a different order. His or her blood sugar soon drops low, but the liver does not release much of its glycogen because emotional or physical triggers have not been pulled.

The ditch digger, whose glucose and glycogen bank account may have been overdrawn, eats with gusto. However, the desk worker (who may eat with equal gusto) may still have a good bank balance of glycogen in the liver. Due to this reserve, much of his or her food intake is turned into fat and stored in fat cells.

Here's a fact to remember if you want to lose weight: Unless you perform some appreciable physical work or exercise not long after your intake of food, you may have surplus calories, another name for fat, for storage in the most conspicuous places.

HUNGER AND EXERCISE

Appetite is stepped up with greater exercise, admits Dr. Jean Mayer.[2] However, this does not nullify the value of increased physical activity. It only explains the body's constant striving to keep weight relatively constant, to keep from burning away its substance when called upon to exert itself beyond customary limits. Such adjustments of calorie intake and output have limitations even in a normal individual.

Rat experiments by Mayer and associates at Harvard some years ago established a new set of ground rules and a more specific answer to this issue. Animals that exercised from one to two hours daily ate slightly less than unexercised rats. Rats exercised for two hours or more increased their food intake up to the end of their activity and endurance. Then the exhausted animals ate less and lost weight.

Mayer observes that neither extreme, minimum activity nor exhaustion, is normal and that *low levels of exercise do not necessarily cause an increase of food intake.*[3]

However, physical inactivity has been discovered to contribute more to developing obesity than eating too much.

James H. Greene, M.D., of Iowa City, Iowa, demonstrated this principle with a study of 200 patients. Obesity began in them when physical activity stopped short because of drastic life changes: a new occupation, going blind, a serious accident involving fractures, or some other cause for becoming sedentary. Becoming physically inactive did not bring about a decrease in the amount of food eaten.[4]

INACTIVITY ENCOURAGES OBESITY

A study of Massachusetts high school girls by Drs. Mayer and Mary Louise Johnson some years ago revealed that inactivity contributes far more to obesity than relative overeating. A survey of the food intake of obese and normal girls matched by age and height disclosed two distinct categories of obese subjects: (1) the super heavyweights, who ate slightly fewer calories but exercised far less than the normal weights and spent four times more hours watching television; and (2) a small segment of outgoing, cheerful, obese girls who out-ate the normal-weight girls and exercised as much. Exercise made them more muscular and less plump-looking than the sedentary obese girls.[5]

Two later studies by Mayer produced additional significant

findings. In the first, obese and non-obese children of the same age and social status were filmed while swimming and playing tennis and volleyball. Heavyweights moved only a fraction as much as the normal weights and expended far less energy.

In the second study, obese and normal-weight boys matched by age, height, and social and economic status at a summer camp were carefully observed. Physical activity was mandatory for all. Normal-weight boys ate more and gained poundage, while the obese boys ate only slightly more and lost weight.[6]

EXERCISE HELPS THE OBESE LOSE FASTER

In one respect, obese persons have an advantage over the moderately overweight: a greater potential for melting off unwanted weight.

While exercising, the obese expend more energy than normal weights because of impaired and cumbersome movements and excessive poundage, says Mayer. If fed as usual, the obese will burn off much more body fat than the moderately overweight.

Even a 20 percent overweight individual can lose more poundage than the normal weight performing the same physical activity, since accumulated fat makes the exercise more clumsy and inefficient.[7]

So if you are 20 percent or more overweight and exercise vigorously and regularly, you have everything to lose (pounds) and something to gain: a sense of accomplishment, greater self-esteem, and a more slender you. The heavyweight who habitually spends too much time sitting down fails to capitalize on the fat-melting advantage of exercise.

If you are substantially overweight, if you have trouble shedding surplus fat and think that things are stacked against you and life is unfair, you are not paranoid. You are right!

PARADOX ABOUT WEIGHT LOSS

Ironically, today's society, which worships slenderness, tantalizes you with irresistible, high-calorie foods and keeps you from exercising with endless labor-saving devices at work and at home.

Typical is the telephone extension cord, which AT&T claims can save you from walking 70 unnecessary miles a year. Dr. Mayer estimates that this saving of 5,000 calories annually for a 150-pound person means he or she will gain 15 pounds within 10 years. Multiple phones and portable units save even more steps.[8]

The golfer plays eighteen holes and drives around in a battery-powered cart. Weight-loss authorities Richard B. Stuart and Barbara Davis point out the phenomenal sales growth of exercising machines, appliances, and devices. They wryly write that billions of dollars are spent on labor-saving machines, while only millions are being expended for labor-making devices.

Much of the overweight you may be toting around could be attributable to the fact that, as society has shifted from manual labor to machine labor, we haven't learned to lower our calorie intake accordingly. What calories we don't spend, we bank.

Aside from inertia—powerful resistance to doing anything physical about overweight—are these labor-saving devices depriving you of a sleek physique?

1. Electric hedge clippers.

2. Power lawn mower.

3. Tractor-type lawn mower.

4. Snow blower.

5. The remote control TV channel selector.

6. Ready-cut wood for the fireplace.

7. Elevators.

8. Escalators.

9. Airport automatic walkways.

10. The automobile.

11. Electric carving knives, cream whippers, food processors, toothbrushes, and garage-door openers.

FREE THE MECHANICAL SLAVES IN YOUR LIFE

If you are serious about losing weight, liberate your electrical and mechanical slave laborers and launch a do-it-yourself movement. Here are some easy-to-do activities that will whittle you down, just as not doing them has done the opposite:

1. If you already have an additional phone, hurry to the more distant phone to answer calls.

2. Try not to save steps. Take them.

3. Walk. Don't always drive.

4. Walk rapidly, if possible, for thirty minutes or more.

5. Take the stairs, not the elevator, unless you are physically impaired.

6. Walk to work, if the area is safe. (I read about a fellow who walked in a high-crime district and got mugged.)

7. Park a mile or two from work and walk, if the area is safe.

8. Stand as you dress or undress (if your equilibrium is normal).

9. Walk or jog at your desk during breaks and during noon hours.

10. Wash and wax your own car. (Forget about status and pride. Your weight loss program is more important.)

11. Pursue housework and yardwork with great zest, enthusiasm, and energy. Sluggish activity burns fewer calories.

12. Use your legs, not your remote-control TV channel selector.

Several of my patients have lost a half pound to a pound a week just by adding these calorie-spending activities.

Over and above such behavior modifications, you might wish to consider exercises that are most effective in controlling weight. Most published research favors exertion that uses the greatest amount of muscle mass and moves the body for considerable distances with vigor. Richard B. Stuart and Barbara Davis favor running, which they say burns up more fat (stored energy) than push-ups.

THE GREATEST FAT MELTERS

Dr. Grant Gwinup says that stationary bicycling is "the most effective calorie burner," as revealed by his comparative studies.

Don't confuse this person-powered exercise with use of an electrically driven bicycle. Although the body is in motion on the latter, there is little contraction of muscles, and calorie usage is small. *You* are the magical ingredient in using up stored calories—not the electrically powered bike, which has no extra poundage to lose.

Dr. Gwinup says that running and jogging come next in efficient calorie burning. Contrary to popular opinion, swimming is not the best exercise for weight loss, as his comparative experiments show.

Moderately obese healthy young women who wanted to lose weight by daily exercise rather than by dieting were randomly assigned to one of three types of physical activity: brisk walking, stationary bicycle riding, or swimming.

Over some 28 weeks, the test subjects increased their exercise time from 5 to 60 minutes daily. The walkers lost 11 percent of their initial weight, the cyclists, 13 percent, and the swimmers, nothing. In fact, they gained 3 percent.

Why the gain for swimmers?

"I suspect it was because the body's natural defense mechanism against cold is to hoard fat," says Dr. Gwinup. "Eskimos are among the world's fattest people. Polynesians, who spend much time in water, are also fat. Japanese women pearl divers, who swim for many hours daily, are fit but fat."

Additional factors in burning fat are: how strenuously you exercise and for how long, and how much you weigh.

During my appearances on radio and TV talk shows, I am often asked whether or not isometric exercises contribute much to weight loss. In isometrics, you benefit from muscle contractions but not from total body movement and turnover of large amounts of oxygen. You use various muscles against one another or against an object such as a wall. However, weight loss is almost negligible compared with working large muscle mass and making wholesale body movements.

Most authorities agree that the best fat-melting exercises involve the Big Three of activity: (1) use of large muscle mass, (2) muscle contraction, and (3) gross movement of the body from one place to another.

Bicycle riding, running, and jogging are the best examples of this, according to Dr. Gwinup. Such exercises—not for the soft and sedentary without proper pre-conditioning—are especially effective if sustained for thirty minutes or more. They are called aerobic exercises because they utilize great amounts of oxygen and benefit the respiratory system, heart, and arteries.

Climbing stairs is one of the better aerobic exercises and a great fat melter, but I hesitate to recommend it because of the accident hazard it presents. A hospital bed is not the best place in the world to lose weight.

Aside from using additional oxygen and stimulating the entire cardiovascular system, aerobic exercise speeds up your metabolism, as Dr. Gwinup mentioned earlier. Also, the fat-burning process goes on for several hours after you quit exercising.

CHOOSE YOUR MOST EFFICIENT CALORIE BURNERS

So that you can maximize results of your exercising, here's a chart listing various physical activities—light, moderate, and heavy—that shows how many calories you burn up per minute in each. The chart is invaluable for another reason: it permits you to select exercises according to your capability and physical condition at this time and shows you which ones burn off the most fat per minute expended.

The following figures cannot be precise to the greatest degree because your specific weight is a key factor, too.

If you have been sedentary or ill for a long time, and are overweight by more than 20 percent, start your exercise program slowly after getting an okay from your doctor.

TABLE 1
AVERAGE ENERGY EXPENDITURE DURING RECREATIONAL ACTIVITIES*

Light Exercise 4 calories/ minute	Moderate Exercise 7 calories/minute	Heavy Exercise 10 calories/minute
Dancing (slow step) Gardening (light) Golf Table tennis Volleyball Walking (3 mi./hr.)	Badminton (singles) Cycling (9.5 mi./hr.) Dancing (fast step) Gardening (heavy) Stationary cycling (moderately) Swimming (30 yd./min.) Tennis (singles) Walking (4.5 mi./hr.)	Calisthenics (vigorous) Climbing stairs (up & down) Cycling (12 mi./hr.) Handball, paddleball, squash Jogging Skipping rope Stationary cycling (quickly) Stationary jogging Swimming (40 yd./min.)

*Values are for gross energy expenditure.
Reproduced with permission from Stuart, R.B. and Davis, B. (1972), Slim chance in a fat world: Behavioral control of obesity (professional edition). Champaign, IL: Research Press.

DON'T DO TOO MUCH TOO SOON

There are three dangers in over-enthusiasm and over-zealousness too early: (1) a physical accident; (2) exhaustion and disinclination to continue; and (3) sore muscles, cramps, and, when seeing little or no immediate weight loss, a feeling of "Is this all worthwhile?"

It is. If at first you have to slow down or reduce your exercising, do so but continue. Make exercising a daily habit. If you've had a track record of quitting because you lost little or no weight, you may not have exercised long enough.

One of Dr. Gwinup's experiments illustrates this point. Eleven obese women increased their time walking each day for a year or more. (They remained on their usual diet.)

Not one of them was able to lose until she began walking *more than thirty minutes a day!*

Maybe you haven't worked up to thirty-plus minutes of daily exercise and have stopped just short of losing!

Dr. Gwinup states that the women averaged a twenty-two-pound weight loss and maintained this for a year or more. When your weight plateaus, increase the amount of exercise and you will lose again. You won't reach your weight-loss goal overnight, but you will reach it with continued effort and patience.

Gwinup warns against losing too much too fast. Be content with dropping a pound a week, he advises. If you do it faster, you'll be losing only water and muscle, as well as "important minerals and other nutrients essential to your health."

For those who want to win at weight loss, patience is not only a virtue, it's a necessity. Combine your exercise with the behavioral techniques for cutting down on foods mentioned in the last chapter.

You pay a penalty in terms of extra exercise if you eat extras to boost your morale for an exercise program.

How much? Skim over items on the following chart to learn this.

HOW TO MAKE YOURSELF WANT TO EXERCISE

How can you motivate yourself to exercise and eat less or at least the same amount? By negatives or positives. It's dealer's choice.

Psychologists find some motivational values for heavy-weights in standing naked in front of a full-length mirror and saying something like:

"If I gain anymore, I'll need a wider mirror," or, "I'll soon have to pay double for an airline ticket," or, "Soon I'll have to weigh myself on a truck scale," or, "Unless I lose this blubber, I'll have to trade my dressmaker for a tentmaker," or, "I lost a pound last week. What's so little against so much?"

Why not reverse the last statement to, "I lost a pound last

TABLE 2
ENERGY EQUIVALENTS OF FOOD CALORIES EXPRESSED IN MINUTES OF ACTIVITY

FOOD	CALORIES	Walking*	Riding bicycle†	Swimming‡	Running#	Reclining¶
		min.	min.	min.	min.	min.
Apple, large	101	19	12	9	5	78
Bacon, 2 strips	96	18	12	9	5	74
Banana, small	88	17	11	8	4	68
Beans, green 1 c.	27	5	3	2	1	21
Beer, 1 glass	114	22	14	10	6	88
Bread and butter	78	15	10	7	4	60
Cake, 1/12, 2-layer	356	68	43	32	18	274
Carbonated beverage, 1 glass	106	20	13	9	5	82
Carrot, raw	42	8	5	4	2	32
Cereal dry, 1/2 c., with milk and sugar	200	38	24	18	10	154
Cheese, cottage, 1 Tbsp.	27	5	3	2	1	21
Cheese, Cheddar, 1 oz.	111	21	14	10	6	85
Chicken, fried, 1/2 breast	232	45	28	21	12	178
Chicken, "TV" dinner	542	104	66	48	28	417
Cookie, plain, 148/lb.	15	3	2	1	1	12
Cookie, chocolate chip	51	10	6	5	3	39
Doughnut	151	29	18	13	8	116
Egg, fried	110	21	13	10	6	85
Egg, boiled	77	15	9	7	4	59
French dressing, 1 Tbsp.	59	11	7	5	3	45

Halibut steak, ¼ lb.	205	39	25	18	11	158
Ham, 2 slices	167	32	20	15	9	128
Ice cream, ⅙ qt.	193	37	24	17	10	148
Ice cream soda	255	49	31	23	13	196
Ice milk, ⅙ qt.	144	28	18	13	7	111
Gelatin, with cream	117	23	14	10	6	90
Malted milk shake	502	97	61	45	26	386
Mayonnaise, 1 Tbsp.	92	18	11	8	5	71
Milk, 1 glass	166	32	20	15	9	128
Milk, skim, 1 glass	81	16	10	7	4	62
Milk shake	421	81	51	38	22	324
Orange, medium	68	13	8	6	4	52
Orange juice, 1 glass	120	23	15	11	6	92
Pancake with syrup	124	24	15	11	6	95
Peach, medium	46	9	6	4	2	35
Peas, green, ½ c.	56	11	7	5	3	43
Pie, apple, ⅙	377	73	46	34	19	290
Pie, raisin, ⅙	437	84	53	39	23	336
Pizza, cheese, ⅛	180	35	22	16	9	138
Pork chop, loin	314	60	38	28	16	242
Potato chips, 1 serving	108	21	13	10	6	83
Sandwiches						
Club	590	113	72	53	30	454
Hamburger	350	67	43	31	18	269
Roast beef with gravy	430	83	52	38	22	331
Tuna fish salad	278	53	34	25	14	214
Sherbet, ⅙ qt.	177	34	22	16	9	136
Shrimp, French fried	180	35	22	16	9	138
Spaghetti, 1 serving	396	76	48	35	20	305

TABLE 2 CONTINUED
ENERGY EQUIVALENTS OF FOOD CALORIES EXPRESSED IN MINUTES OF ACTIVITY

| | | | ACTIVITY | | | |
| | | | Riding | | | |
FOOD	CALORIES	Walking*	bicycle†	Swimming‡	Running#	Reclining¶
		min.	min.	min.	min.	min.
Steak, T-bone	235	45	29	21	12	181
Strawberry shortcake	400	77	49	36	21	308

*Energy cost of walking for 70-kg. individual = 5.2 calories per minute at 3.5 m.p.h.
†Energy cost of riding bicycle = 8.2 calories per minute.
‡Energy cost of swimming = 11.2 calories per minute.
#Energy cost of running = 19.4 calories per minute.
¶Energy cost of reclining = 1.3 calories per minute.
Konishi, F.: Food energy equivalents of various activities. Copyright the American Dietetic Association. Reprinted
by permission from JOURNAL OF THE AMERICAN DIETETIC ASSOCIATION. Vol. 46: 186, 1965.

week. Great! I'll do it again this week,'' or, ''Every time I lose a pound, I'm healthier and happier, and have more self-respect because I'm managing my overweight. It is no longer managing me,'' or, ''My clothes fit a little better now. It won't be long before I'll fit comfortably in a smaller size.''

My patients get amazing reinforcement from losing weight and showing better health, as indicated by my physical checkups and lab reports: more favorable HDL cholesterol in ratio to LDL, lower triglycerides, declining blood pressure, and improved blood-sugar readings.

It's never too late to participate in regular physical activity to lose weight and gain health ''Brownie points.'' In an experimental program, Dr. Herbert DeVries, of the University of Southern California School of Medicine,[9] supervised a moderate, 15-minute daily exercise routine for men from 52 to 88 years old. Within several months, participants lost their flab; they developed 35 percent more breathing capacity, a 30 percent increase in ability to deliver oxygen to cells, greater ability to sleep soundly, relief from nervous tension, anger, frustration, aggression, and hostility, along with well-being and more youthful appearance.

REINFORCE YOURSELF WITH THE BUDDY SYSTEM

It was easier for all the men to participate regularly because so many of their friends also were involved. The ''buddy system'' is one of the most effective reinforcements to seek. The presence of many others trying to lose weight makes a health club a good place to work out.

My patients often find an exercise partner at home, at the office, or in school. They reinforce one another in dieting as well as in exercising.

There may be times when you need support as an alcoholic needs backing by a fellow AA member. Make a pact with your mate or friend. Set goals together for weight loss. With such reinforcement, you can only win, and, as you win, you will lose.

14 | The Setpoint— How to Beat It

Psychologists tell us that we have a setpoint something like a thermostat that controls storage of body fat. Since we are all unique and different, some of us have a setting for a low amount of fat storage, others for a high amount.

Perhaps the setpoint theory explains why many obese people claim to eat very little and, yet, gain very much. As a matter of fact, a survey by weight authority Dr. Albert Stunkard makes this very point.

Stunkard and associates observed eaters of all weights, shapes, and sizes in fast-food establishments serving standardized portions: pizza parlors and snack bars.[1] They found that those who were 30 percent overweight ate about the same quantities as leaner individuals. However, what the study did not cover was how many other fast-food establishments the observed persons had just visited.

One of the most extreme examples of a person with a malfunctioning setpoint was ponderous Robert Earl Hughes, of Monticello, Missouri. At the ripe young age of thirty-two, Robert died at 1,041 pounds—a weight that hurried him into a vast grave and into the pages of Ripley's *Believe It Or Not*.

The basic purpose of the body setpoint is survival: to store enough fat to keep us alive in the event of starvation. Apparently, it is difficult for some of us to lose weight because the body cannot distinguish between a voluntary effort at weight reduction and the threat of starvation.

A CLOSEUP ON THE SETPOINT

A popular theory of how the setpoint works against the heavy person was devised by Rockefeller University obesity researchers Jules Hirsch, Irving Faust, and Rudolph Leibel. They believe the fat cells themselves, through the central nervous system, give the signal to overeat.[2]

Fat cells of the obese are often two to two and a half times as large as those of normal-weight persons, indicating that the biochemical system regulating fat-cell size has gone awry, say these researchers.

As a person gains weight, his or her metabolism speeds up dramatically, lavishly using excess calories to consume food. In the weight-loss phase, the opposite happens. The metabolic machinery perversely uses far fewer calories in consuming food. It zealously protects the status quo.

The Rockefeller University team also discovered why people have difficulty losing weight in certain areas—for example, the hips in women. Leibel explains that fat cells have two types of receptors on their surfaces: alpha, which accumulate fat, and beta, which help break down fat. When alpha receptors predominate, fat storage takes place faster than breakdown.

Unfortunately, these researchers have no quick fix for too many alpha receptors in specific areas. They still need to know more about the conduct of receptors and fat cells.

Meanwhile, the best formula for outwitting the setpoint is slowly reducing your intake of calories and increasing your energy output (exercise).

Energy output actually breaks down into three parts: (1) basal metabolism (how fast you burn up food in your cells at resting level), (2) thermogenesis (energy in the form of heat given off above the metabolic rate at resting state), and, of course, (3) physical activity.[3]

Put in simplest terms, basal metabolism relates to efficiency of the thyroid gland. Two major factors contributing to thermogenesis are food intake and exposure to temperatures below body temperature. Food-induced thermogenesis comes in two separate forms: obligatory and regulatory. Obligatory are the energy costs of digesting, absorbing, and converting nutrients for use and storage. Regulatory are the ways of dissipating energy: physical and mental activity.

BIOGRAPHY OF BROWN FAT

Still another critical part of thermogenesis is brown fat, a special kind of adipose tissue that collects below the neck and extends down the back. All men and women are not created equal so far as amount of brown fat is concerned. Persons who have inherited a small amount have more difficulty staying slender than those who were born with a good supply. Persons whose brown fat functions inefficiently are as bad off as those who were short-changed.

Just what does brown fat do?

It helps convert deposits of the usual body fat into heat and dissipate it. Young and adult genetically obese animals have been found to have defective brown fat function. Researchers now conclude that this flaw is a *cause* of obesity in animals not a *result*.[4]

What causes brown fat to get into the act?

Some researchers have found that parts of the brain—mainly the hypothalamus, which governs the sympathetic nervous system's response to food intake and to the temperature of the body's environment—trigger the action of brown fat, whose mitochondria (power houses) are especially designed to generate heat.

Lean persons possess the most effective brown-fat heat production ability and decreased metabolic efficiency. When food is restricted, heat generation in brown fat is suppressed while metabolic efficiency increases.

Several studies show that faulty brown-fat heat production is obesity-associated in different types of grossly fat animals.

Once obesity develops, whether in animals or in human beings, another factor complicates thermogenesis, says Dr. Jean

Mayer: the insulating blanket of fat that blocks the dissipating of heat.[5]

One of the strategies for revving up thermogenesis for weight reduction is using drugs such as ephedrine, a known stimulant of this process. I do not favor this method.

A study in the use of ephedrine to stimulate thermogenic responsiveness revealed a significant reduction in mean body weight after a four and a twelve week treatment: 2.5 and 5.5 kg, respectively. This translates into roughly 5½ and 12 pounds, respectively. The researchers conclude that ephedrine may be useful in the treatment of obesity.[6]

T-3: A HELPFUL FACTOR

One of the best known stimulators of thermogenesis is thyroid hormone. When the thyroid gland is functioning normally, you are usually warm and have warm hands and feet in a moderately warm room where the temperature is 25 degrees or less below body temperature.

However, when your thyroid function is deficient, you and your extremities are cold. Then I would prescribe natural, desiccated thyroid, which almost always boosts body temperature, as demonstrated by the Barnes Basal Temperature Test.

An experiment described not long ago in *Clinical Endocrinology* showed the effectiveness of a single thyroid hormone (T3) in stimulating thermogenesis and inducing weight loss.[7]

Four groups of obese individuals matched by Body Mass Index were placed on different, three-week, starvation diets (480 Kcal) followed by an eight-week, low-Kcal diet (1,008 Kcal)—20 percent protein and 40 percent carbohydrate, with or without low doses of triiodothyronine (T3).

Groups 1 and 2 received a placebo. Groups 3 and 4 were administered a low dose of T3 (20 micrograms) twice daily. Patients taking T3 showed a greater weight loss than any others.

During semi-starvation, patients on the low-protein diet (33 grams) had a lower nitrogen reserve than those on a high-protein regime. The researchers concluded that T3 therapy helps cause weight loss in patients on a low calorie diet, although nitrogen balance was upset on a low-protein diet.

Therefore, if you and your doctor decide that T3 therapy is worth a try, remember that at least 66 grams of protein along with your low-calorie diet should keep your nitrogen supply in balance.

Probably the greatest influence on weight loss is prolonged, tiring physical exercise, which not only speeds up and sustains higher metabolism but, in the process, increases thermogenesis.

So far as heat generation is concerned, thyroid hormones have a direct and indirect effect on energy production. An article in *Clinical Endocrinology-Metabolism* states that thyroid hormones directly affect the basal (resting) metabolic rate in man and have been shown to influence heat generation through inefficient metabolic pathways.[8]

Thyroid hormones help you to increase body-heat production to keep body temperature higher than that of the surrounding air. They even exert an indirect influence on the thermogenesis in brown fat.

Animal studies reveal that variations in food intake and physical activity regulate energy balance. This dual control may help explain why certain people seem to put on weight more rapidly than others.

Another clue as to why some individuals become obese is a little-known function of insulin, as a moderator of how much body heat is increased following eating. Most of us only know of insulin's role in regulating blood sugar.[9]

When there's too little insulin and resistance to it, the body decreases dissipation of fat by means of heat. This means you gain weight and increase your tendency to add even more unwanted poundage.

FUEL BURNING NOT EQUAL IN ALL CELLS

If you ever consider your metabolism, you may think that burning of fuels in all the cells of your body is uniform. Not so.

It differs in various parts of the body. It is particularly varying in the obese.[10]

Recent studies show that metabolism in the fatty deposits of super heavyweights is more sluggish than in other types of tissue. One research project reveals that fat cells in the area of the thighs are larger than in the abdominal region. Lipids are mobilized more slowly and synthesized faster in the thighs than in the abdomen.

When you are on a fast, fat is mobilized slower and synthesized more rapidly in all the fat collection areas—but especially in the abdomen. If you are obese, there are also regional differences in hormonal regulation of fat metabolism. Insulin works best in fat removal in the thighs. However, catecholamines are most effective for this purpose in the abdominal region. Catecholamines are secretions of the adrenal gland, including norepinephrine and dopamine, which influence the central nervous system.[11]

These findings explain why fat accumulates more readily in certain areas and also why certain fat areas are so resistant to slimming. They relate to discoveries of the Hirsch-Faust-Leibel team at Rockefeller University that a higher population of alpha receptors in fat cells encourages storage of fat, while a higher population of beta receptors dissipates fat.

Among many trail-blazing discoveries made by Dr. Hirsch in more than twenty years of research on human fat cells is that obese individuals weighing twice as much as lean test subjects carried three times as much body fat.

You will appreciate Dr. Hirsch's findings if you consider fat cells as microscopic, flexible, rubber bags. As they inflate with more and more fat, you inflate with them. The obese have as many as three times more fat cells than the slender subjects —75 billion to 27 billion in one measurement. Although we never lose fat cells, they can reduce in size. In the obese, the number of fat cells may even increase.

As this chapter has disclosed, there are several approaches to outflanking the stubborn setpoint that wants to keep you plump, if not obese. But the best method for outmaneuvering it is to approach dieting slowly. A crash program seems to alert the setpoint to resist even more resolutely. A moderate dietary intake coupled with a vigorous, daily, sweat-creating exercise program will fire up your body heat to burn fat faster.

My best successes with obese patients have come from the above two-pronged program after eliminating the many hidden causes for overweight mentioned in Chapter 1: low thyroid function, Candida albicans, low blood sugar, heavy-metals intoxication, and food and/or environmental sensitivities and allergies.

15 | Three Squares Could Make You Round

In a weight-control diet, much is made of what to eat and how much, and little about when and how often. Increasing evidence indicates that the latter factors may be of critical importance, too.

Let me illustrate with a story about one of my new patients, a portly male.

"I slash my calories by skipping an occasional meal," he told me during our first appointment. "I'll skip breakfast, lunch, or dinner."

"How many pounds have you lost in the last several weeks?" I asked.

Randy grinned sheepishly.

"I gained five pounds."

I felt for him. What agony he must have undergone, skipping meals for which his body was crying out, and then the payoff: disastrous results.

One of the worst aspects of meal skipping is that would-be weight losers usually skip the wrong meals: breakfast or lunch. I told Randy that if he insisted on skipping any meal, it should be dinner, because few individuals exercise or work physically enough after this meal to burn some of it off.

I also explained that many obese persons skip meals, as one well-designed study shows. The heavyweights are noted for omitting meals needed most to power them through the workday. Many of them also have their dinner at odd hours, compared with normal-weight individuals—often late at night.

BENEFITS OF MANY SMALL MEALS

Some years ago, I read several studies that revealed that many small meals daily can help you lose weight more effectively than the same number of calories in three meals daily.

I make patients aware that three squares could make them round. Although there is not unanimous agreement on the subject, several reputable researchers have discovered that if test persons eat six or seven meals daily with the same caloric values as the three meals they normally eat, they usually lose weight.

On this basis, I have put sixty-three overweight patients on the numerous-small-meals diet with a rewarding success rate. Fifty-two of them have lost one-half pound to a pound a week; on the same number of calories in three meals, they were gaining one-quarter of a pound to a half pound weekly.

Such results are more than a little encouraging, because these patients did nothing else to contribute to their steady weight loss, not even additional exercise.

A second benefit from the frequent-feeding plan is keeping the blood-sugar level normal, which provides energy for work and other activities and helps fend off emotional ailments such as depression. A feeling of satiation with six or seven small meals keeps my overweight patients from binges.

I have urged them to experiment with the frequent-feeding plan. Possibly even five or four feedings would give them desired results. Some have lost appreciable poundage even on four daily meals. However, most of them do better on five, six, or seven small daily feedings.

Biochemist Richard A. Passwater, author of the best-selling book *Supernutrition*, tells of physical benefits from many small meals. In an experiment he permitted laboratory animals to eat as often as they wished, and they thrived. Passwater recommends that we eat five or six times daily to keep from overloading or overworking our complicated digestion and transport system. Frequent feedings put less stress on reserves of organs and the heart, he says.[1]

HOW TO MAKE THE THREE-MEAL SYSTEM WORK

Although each mini meal need not be balanced, there should be a daily balance. The three-square-meal system is not calculated to take off weight unless you follow the principle of a hearty breakfast, a modest lunch, and a spare dinner. It is well to remember that the three-daily-meals system was not necessarily planned to feed us well, to consider our stomach, digestion, and assimilation system—or metabolism, for that matter. Its objective was to accommodate workers in the Industrial Age. That it did and little more.

The three-meal system seems designed to add unwanted weight. Most individuals eat a light breakfast: juice, toast, and coffee—then a slightly more generous lunch and a heavy dinner.

"But I can't eat breakfast," many individuals complain to me.

"Yes, you can," I reply. "Just skip dinner for several days, and soon you will have an appetite for breakfast, a good nutritious one."

Actually, you are in control. Your eating habits are not in the driver's seat unless you abdicate your control.

REVEALING EXPERIMENTS

Not long ago, I stumbled upon some fascinating experiments demonstrating that eating the heaviest meals nearest the time of highest daily activity contributes to weight loss. These were related by Mark Bricklin, executive editor of *Prevention* magazine, in his book, *Lose Weight Naturally*.

Scientists at the University of Minnesota's Chronobiology Laboratories made some interesting findings connected with feeding of mice. These small, experimental animals, which are most active during hours of darkness, were fed only at the start of their activity phase. They came out weighing less than when they were fed by the early morning light, a period when usually they are inactive.

So much for mice? What about people?

The same research group performed the same basic experiment with seven human beings. Of course, this one was adapted to man's usual daylight pattern of activity.

The human subjects ate one 2,000-calorie meal as either a breakfast or dinner. This was their total day's nutrition. After a week, the individuals who had eaten the 2,000 calories for breakfast all lost an average of 2.5 pounds more than those who ate their 2,000 calories at dinner. As a matter of fact, a few of the latter group lost a slight amount, but most of them gained.

Next, the same scientists designed an experiment that more closely reflected typical feeding patterns. Test subjects were free to eat whatever they wanted and as much as they pleased. The only ground rule imposed upon them was that they had to take in all their calories at breakfast or dinnertime.

The same individuals who had eaten their way through the previous experiments endured this one for six weeks and then were carefully checked. Those who ate a heavy breakfast averaged a weight loss of 1.4 pounds more per week.

IT PAYS TO CHANGE LONG-STANDING EATING HABITS

A more recent experiment produced similar results. Used as test subjects were 595 overweight patients in "reasonably good health."

As reported in the *Journal of the Louisiana State Medical Society*, the patients were requested to change long-standing eating habits, particularly desisting from a heavy dinner. Instead they were to have a heavy breakfast, a moderate lunch, and a light dinner. The number of calories in this drastic feeding pattern change was to remain the same.[2]

Although all patients did not adhere religiously to the program's timing, the ideal plan was to eat an early breakfast, lunch in mid-morning and dinner at noon (but not later than 3 p.m.). One key rule was that patients should have at least an 8½-hour interval between their last food intake and going to sleep.

Every patient who followed instructions conscientiously lost weight. The breakfast-only eaters averaged an appreciable 10-pound weight loss per month. The breakfast-lunch-dinner eaters averaged a weight loss of five to six pounds per month. Not one person in the experiment experienced a negative side effect.

Individuals who shed from twenty to thirty pounds during the program showed an increase in their hemoglobin level. The good news for diabetic patients was that those who dropped thirty or more pounds showed normalized blood sugar. Hypothyroid patients who lost at least thirty pounds showed a reduced need for thyroid supplementation.

Although this was only a preliminary study and lacked a control group, the signs are favorable for you if you are willing to modify your eating habits to conform with patterns of this study.

Based on several earlier experiments, I have long put my most stubborn weight-loss cases on a regime similar to that reported in the *Journal of the Louisiana State Medical Society*.

My patients have scored phenomenal weight loss with it. Here is what I suggest for their eating.

"Eat breakfast like Henry VIII; eat lunch sparingly—as if you have to pick up the bill—and eat dinner as if you're a pauper."

It works, and my patients prefer it to turning themselves into accountants with endless, burdensome calorie counting.

16 | Grapefruit, Yak Milk, Brown Rice, and You

Few, if any, diets consider body rhythms. Few diets gear food intake to the period of highest energy expenditure, as covered in the last chapter.

Most weight-control regimes ignore *when* food is eaten and *how fast*. They play a strict numbers game: keeping intake of calories below expended calories.

Some are ineffective. Others are ineffective and hazardous to your health. In this tradition, every month or so somebody comes up with a new wonder diet featuring a single, particular food or food group.

At first it seems to work wonders, but, after a while, you wonder if it works. Who needs another Marvelous Mushroom Diet, Great Australian Hothouse Cucumber Diet, or the Fabulous Fermented Yak Milk Diet?

Not you, if you are serious about shedding surplus weight permanently. Any regime that features one food or food group is suspect because it is too unbalanced to sustain good health and too monotonous to follow.

Can you imagine eating only—or mainly—grapefruit, brown rice, or Australian Hothouse cucumbers for the rest of your life, or drinking only fermented yak milk until the end?

Neither can your taste buds, your stomach, or the rest of your body, so the inevitable thing is that you will eventually gain back all you lost.

If you experience the ups and downs of appreciable weight fluctuation often enough, you can seriously injure your health.

This yo-yo pattern, which Dr. Jean Mayer calls the "rhythm method of girth control," is a body stress that can lop years off your life expectancy. Losing pounds and keeping them off, on the other hand, usually elongates the lifespan.

Weight-control authority Richard B. Stuart finds that weight fluctuations contribute more stress to the arteries than remaining overweight.[1] Further, animal experiments reveal that repeated attempts to diet away surplus poundage deranges metabolism to such an extent that it is increasingly difficult to lose weight even on a severely restricted diet.

Some years ago, doctors at Michael Reese Hospital and Medical Center (Chicago), alarmed at the rash of quick and "easy weight-loss" regimes, sounded a protest against such diets: the macrobiotic, the grapefruit, the low-carbohydrate, and the liquid protein in particular.[2]

Their imbalance and ineffectiveness troubled these physicians, but not as much as their hazard to health.

"I don't even like the word diet," says world-famous cardiologist Ruth Pick, M.D. "The first question a doctor hears when he or she prescribes a diet is, 'How long will I have to stay on it?'[3] Well, of course, as soon as a dieter stops dieting, the weight comes right back."

Dr. Pick recommends establishing new eating habits to remove weight permanently. Patients quickly become disillusioned with a sensible, balanced reducing diet because it doesn't bring about instant weight loss.

Observing that dieters despair when they see little or no weight loss in several weeks, Dr. Pick explains why fat seems reluctant to depart.

". . . When fat leaves the body, the shell—the fat cell—remains. Weight loss or gain doesn't change the *number* of fat cells. At first, as fat leaves, the cells fill with water, so no change is noticeable.

"Eventually, the water also leaves, and the cells shrink. Unfortunately, before that happens, the dieter often gives up hope and returns to old, poor eating habits."

Dr. Pick recommends not giving up hope.

"The average American is used to eating much more than he needs. He feels hungry on less, because his stomach has learned to expect more. If you reduce the amount you eat, you'll stop feeling hungry after about three weeks, when you've become used to less food. Of course, you must retain a nutritionally well-balanced diet while you reduce the number of calories."

Several Michael Reese Hospital doctors admit that occasional fasting won't hurt healthy adults, but it can't substitute for a steady, low-calorie diet.[4]

If you eat a lot one day and fast the next, you cheat your body of nutrition. There are substances needed by the body that can't be stored in time of feast to cover times of famine. So a big meal one day and no meals the next really don't balance out.[5]

Fasting is dangerous for some individuals, agrees pediatrician Dr. Lynne Levitsky—particularly in children in whom it can cause hypoglycemia and possibly a resultant seizure.[6]

"Even in the healthy adult, fasting is a punishment. Sooner or later, you fall back—right into a chocolate creme pie."

Relative to the macrobiotic diet, which calls for progressively more food restriction until the individual eats nothing but brown rice with tea, Dr. Levitsky says:

"It's a disaster nutritionally, and the insidious thing about it is that the rice fills you up, so you may be starving but not feel hungry!"

Then there's more bad news, the grapefruit or Mayo Diet, which keeps the Mayo Clinic frantic denying authorship or support.

THE IMPOTENT GRAPEFRUIT

Michael Reese endocrinologist Murray J. Favus, M.D., comments on it:

"The premise is that grapefruit has an enzyme that breaks down fat faster, so that you can eat a lot, and the grapefruit will keep you slim. Well, the body breaks down enzymes on their way to the stomach. If grapefruit does have such an enzyme, it's destroyed before it can do anything."[7]

So much for the tasty but impotent grapefruit.

Low-carbohydrate diets get the frown from Dr. Favus. "Diets that manipulate weight by denying the body one kind of fuel, can't fool the body."

"For example, the central nervous system needs carbohydrates to function," explains Dr. Leslie Sandlow, gastroenterologist and deputy vice president of Michael Reese. "If it doesn't get them, it takes muscle mass (protein) and turns it into carbohydrate. You can have a lot of fat on your body without eating any fat. Your body makes the conversion for you."[8]

The idea is not to use gimmicks, but to get to the heart of the matter—good nutrition that at the same time slowly eases off poundage.

Vegetarianism is an excellent weight-loss regime, if certain precautions are taken, the Michael Reese doctors indicate. Sufficient protein must be supplied, and can be if enough rice and beans are included. Vitamin supplements are needed as well—particularly vitamin B-12, which is lacking in vegetarian foods.[9]

The major benefit from a vegetarian diet is that it is low in fat, and you can eat more and be satisfied with fewer calories.

WHY YOU SHOULD EAT MORE SLOWLY

Over and above a quality diet as a factor in weight loss is a manner of eating that lessens the intake of calories. Eat more slowly; chew your food to permit digestive juices in your mouth and throat to do their work, but, most of all, to extend your eating time for a meal or even a snack to as much as twenty-five minutes, the time it takes for you to get the feeling that "I've had enough."

Rapid eaters usually consume more food than necessary because they do not give enough time for nature's check system to work.

Stuart has a method of slowing down eaters from a sprint to a walk. (I have used it effectively for scores of overweight patients.) Stop eating shortly after you've started your meal. Just put your knife, fork, or spoon down on the plate for several minutes. This practice does two favorable things. It shows you that you are in control of your compulsively fast eating. The food no longer controls you—a satisfying feeling. Second, you decelerate your eating, he says.[10]

Stuart adds one more rule. Chew and swallow the food in your mouth before adding more. Put your fork or spoon on the edge of the plate, once the food is in your mouth. Don't pick up your utensil again until you have swallowed the food in your mouth.

Dr. Jean Mayer agrees that slowing down the eating process brings favorable results, giving the body's natural reactions the time to transmit the feeling of satiation.[11]

I use a form of the Stuart system with some overweight patients by suggesting that they eat by the clock, that they time themselves and their eating of a typical meal at their usual speed.

It didn't surprise me that the initial timing of some 130 overweight patients ranged from as little as 5 minutes to as much as 12 minutes.

Next I had them extend their eating time for the identical meal to twenty-five minutes. In most instances, they felt satisfied and began cutting down calories in each elongated meal.

Time *yourself*. You will probably discover that you're in the five-to-twelve minute range. Then, begin to eat slowly and lose weight. Remember that haste makes waist.

THE HOME APPLIANCE THAT MAKES YOU OVERWEIGHT

One particular home appliance does more to add weight to you than any other. No, it's not the refrigerator. The one I'm referring to speeds up your eating and hurries you to the refrigerator or the pantry for more ammo.

It's your television set that diverts you from realizing how much you're eating, and how fast. High-tension dramas, especially, rev up your eating tempo and increase your stress level, which interferes with your digestion.

A recent survey of obesity and television viewing in nearly 7,000 children and adolescents shows the insidious influence of TV. In three different groups, it was clearly established that there is an association between the time spent watching TV and obesity. Researchers determined that in the twelve-to-seventeen-year-old group, obesity increased by 2 percent for each additional daily hour of television watching.

Whatever your age, television adds unwanted blubber in four ways: (1) by speeding up your eating; (2) by influencing you to eat more than you need; (3) by persuading you to eat calorie-dense, junk foods; and (4) by gluing you to the chair for hours, keeping you from being physically active and burning up calories.

Granted the subtle and pervasive influence of TV on food intake and your need to decide to eat or not to eat before the tube, you have another equally basic decision to make: which type of diet to follow—balanced, high-protein, low-protein, high-carbohydrate, low-carbohydrate, high-fat, low-fat, or some combination of ingredients, and, above all, total calories.

A study conducted at the University of Wisconsin in Madison dealt with calories first. It was found that most individuals will lose weight if they set their daily caloric intake below 1,500. Yet certain test subjects with normal thyroid function must slash their calories to 1,000 daily to continue dropping weight.[12]

Richard B. Friedman, M.D., vice chairman, department of medicine and director of the school's Weight Reduction Program, says that most moderately obese patients can't tolerate this diet long enough to reach their ideal weight.

Most sound diet programs give slow and sometimes frustrating results—about a half pound per week—and a whopping majority of patients who endure the program long enough to reach their goal regain everything lost within a year or two.

Dr. Friedman states that almost every diet contributes to some weight loss because it cuts calories below what the body requires to keep weight in balance. However, many diets are boring and rigid—who can stay on them?—and certain ones are definite health hazards.

The ideal weight-loss diet includes a daily protein intake of 56 gm for men and 44 gm for women—about 15 to 20 percent of total calories—and 50 percent carbohydrates (with refined sugar confined to less than 10 percent of calories) and fat the remaining amount—roughly 30 to 35 percent—rather than up to 50 percent as it is now.

Play it safe, Dr. Friedman recommends. Use the moderately low-calorie diets, those containing the recommended daily allowances of carbohydrates, fats, protein, minerals, and vitamins—1,000 to 1,800 calories daily, depending upon your weight.

RATING THE MAJOR DIETS

Here's how Dr. Friedman rates the major diets:

1. The setpoint regime which involves lowering your setpoint is not a proved method. Even in animal experiments, it is far from conclusive. The diet itself—low-calorie, calling for 1,200 to 1,800 calories, depending on your weight—requires moderate exercise. This is laudable and basic, but the program is neither novel nor well tested.

2. A high-carbohydrate diet (mainly with complex carbohydrates and high water content) increases bulk and makes you feel great. Coupled with exercise and behavior modification, this one seems advantageous.

3. The high-fiber diet (35 to 50 mg daily), low in protein and in calories (1,000 to 1,250), supposedly binds fat and protein, giving a feeling of satiation. All the claims for it are not well documented, but added fiber enhances the typical American diet.

4. Low-carbohydrate diets usually are low in fats; due to limited carbohydrates, they can't completely oxidize fats. This causes ketosis, whose common symptoms are dehydration, diarrhea, sodium-depletion, excess blood fats, higher uric acid production, exhaustion, and postural hypertension.

5. The high-protein diet is a good loser, yet is often monotonous and hard to stay with over a protracted period. It usually has a high cholesterol content and is not for persons who have gout, diabetes, or kidney or liver disease, or who are pregnant. Unless a great deal of water is taken with it, the body can't rid itself of ketones, which cause fatigue and bad breath. Sometimes, this diet calls for vitamin and mineral supplements.

6. High-fat diets are among the best-tasting and are the slowest through the digestive system, making persons who eat them feel satisfied for a longer period of time. They could cause increased cholesterol levels and, therefore, may not be safe for individuals with hypercholesterolemia, explains Dr. Friedman.

The Amazing Diet Secret of a Desperate Housewife, stressing fructose, lecithin, and kelp is not scientifically sound and is potentially dangerous, states Dr. Friedman.

The Carbohydrate Craver's Diet (1,100 calories and high in carbohydrates), including tryptophan, supposedly controls hunger. This arouses Dr. Friedman's skepticism.

The Last Best Diet Book offers a 600-to-700-calorie regime that is rigid and hard to adhere to. Worst of all, it is unbalanced, including diet days for protein only and binge days, allowing persons to gorge on 2,000 to 3,000 calories.

Radical macrobiotic diets are not only nutritionally unsound, "self-imposed starvation," but are extremely dangerous, says Dr. Friedman.

Over and above the Friedman evaluations are my analyses of three popular regimes that I have experienced: The Cambridge Plan, the Pritikin Diet, and the Beverly Hills Diet.

The Cambridge Plan centers on dietary powder that comes in many delicious flavors, including the ever-popular chocolate. With approximately 330 calories daily and just 33 grams of protein, I find this plan more than severe in restriction of calories and protein—one step up from fasting.

Even though the plan furnishes all the Recommended Daily Allowances (RDA) for vitamins and minerals, its shortage of protein—high-quality though milk and soy protein are—concerns me. Thirty-three grams of protein is considerably under the RDA of 44 grams for women and 56 grams for men.

It was next to impossible for me to stay on this diet. I felt abused, and my body craved more nourishment.

The Pritikin Permanent Weight Loss Diet, top-heavy in complex carbohydrates—all the raw vegetables you can eat—is a marked improvement over previous Pritikin regimes, offering more variety.

There's also an increase in protein to RDA recommended levels. However, as pointed out earlier (in the stress chapter), stresses demand more protein than the minimum—and who, these days, isn't under stress? Further, this diet omits egg yolks in favor of egg whites; therefore, it also omits lecithin, so imperative for a healthy liver.

This diet represents the Pritikin phobia of saturated fats, some of which are needed to contribute to weight loss. Certainly, the American diet contains too much fat, but most authorities recommend a cutback from 40 percent of the diet to around 30 percent, not a drastic limitation.

An improvement over previous Pritikin plans, this one also features a bagful of fresh vegetables—carrots, celery, radishes—to be crunched and munched all day long.

Although there is some merit in the Pritikin Permanent Weight Loss Plan, there is little, if any, in the Beverly Hills Diet, which provides less than marginal nutrition and offers a great risk to health.

The main part of the diet is day-in and day-out fruit and no appreciable protein until you've sweated out eighteen days. Then on the nineteenth day it's lobster or steak.

The Beverly Hills Diet offers near protein starvation. This unbalanced, illogical regime, violating most rules of good nutrition, contributes to fluid loss and, with this, a deficiency of vitally needed minerals, especially potassium. This contributes to suspenseful, irregular heartbeat, diarrhea, fatigue, and depression, among other hazards.

Imagine the diet's first day—only bananas and pineapple for each meal. Next day you eat papaya and mangoes. The third day, it's papaya and pineapple.

The staggering amount of fructose (fruit sugar) in this diet is frightening in the light of recent findings by the United States Department of Agriculture's Research Section.[13]

Excessive fructose in the presence of copper deficiency, highly prevalent with so many processed foods in the diet, can cause acute heart damage. Biochemists with the U.S. Department of Agriculture's Beltsville, Maryland, research center conducted an experiment with pigs on a high-fructose/low-copper regime and found that their hearts had enlarged to twice the size of animals in the control group.

Aside from possible physical damage that can come from a diet which calls for so much fruit, the day-after-day routine of sweet fruits—bananas, pineapple, papaya, mangoes, and watermelon—is enough to drive you to eat salt straight. I know. I've been there.

Frankly, this monotonous fruit diet almost made me go bananas.

If there are so many negatives among popular diets, are there any positives that contribute to weight reduction and are also well-balanced and safe?

Very few.

That is the subject for the next chapter.

17 | Things Mother Never Told You About Food and Overweight

"**C**rash diets" is the right name for most very low-calorie reducing diets, because if you are Spartan enough to endure them for long enough to lose appreciable poundage, your health and you may, indeed, crash.

The idea is to lose fat, not your life.

Most diet books warn how difficult it is to obtain critical nutrients from so few calories. None, to my knowledge, has spelled out the whole problem and presented a real solution.

Let's be candid. Nutritional values of many, if not most, foods are overstated.

You are being short-changed from the ground up—from depleted soils producing depleted foods, from highly processed foods, and from the abomination of imitation foods.

The best place to begin is at the beginning: the soil. Someone once remarked, "You can't pull a rabbit out of the hat unless you've already put one in it."

This principle applies to the earth, to the crops and harvests of today's giant, profit-motivated agribusiness. Vegetables, fruits, grains, and legumes can only draw out of the soil what is there. No magic will make it possible for the five-ingredient chemical fertilizers of today to replace all of the numerous trace minerals that have been drawn out of the soil by crops.

Despite agribusiness rationalizations, the food values of most farm products are declining, as various studies show. What it all adds up to is that, with inflationary food prices, you are paying much more for much less.

The late William A. Albrecht, Ph.D., while professor of soils and chairman of the Department of Soils at the University of Missouri for decades, discovered through many studies that declining soil fertility is responsible for diminishing ability of crops to synthesize protein.[1]

Within a ten-year period, protein content of alfalfa and corn decreased—the latter from 9.5 to 8.5 percent. Some amino acids normally present—they are components of protein—disappeared entirely.

The same thing is happening to our wheat, Albrecht* stated.

"Because trace elements are deficient, should we not consider some diseases as possible deficiencies coming by way of the soil?"

Albrecht reminds us that we are at the top of the biotic pyramid, supported by and dependent on a base of animals, plants, microbes, and soil, as they are dependent upon us. If this base fails, we suffer deficiencies and cannot synthesize the necessary protein from the elements.

And, now, of particular importance to weight gain:

"Plants can synthesize carbohydrates rapidly from air, rainfall and sunshine with but little help from the soil. By this means, crops pile up bulk and fattening food values rapidly.

"But before their life processes—those operating independently of direct sunshine power—can convert those carbohydrates into amino acids and proteins, they must have help from soil fertility . . .

"As long as crop bulk and animals fattened merely for more weight are the major goals of our agriculture, our thinking to no greater depths will delay the day when we see soil as support and in control of production.

"That a soil may be speedily exploited of its protein-producing power while its capacity for delivery of carbohydrate bulk holds on long afterward, is a potent fact that has not yet been recognized . . . Under such circumstances, we shall con-

*Dr. Albrecht's quotations are from *Natural Food and Farming* magazine and are used with permission of the publishers, Natural Food Associates, of Atlanta, Texas.

tinue to talk of 'buying' and rationing protein supplements instead of accepting the costs of soil treatments to grow them.''

Even studies reported in a U.S. Department of Agriculture book demonstrate the necessity for proper fertilization of soil to raise protein content of crops—corn, in this instance.[2]

University of Illinois researchers grew hybrid corn and Illinois High Protein corn on two kinds of plots—unfertilized ground from which corn had been cropped for almost twenty-five years with nothing returned to the soil and plots that had received lime, rock phosphate, and manure. Crop rotation had been practiced.

Protein content of hybrid corn from unfertilized ground was just 7.32 percent, compared with 10.73 percent on the fertilized plots. Protein content of the Illinois High Protein corn from the same two plots was 13.47 and 20.04 percent respectively.

In a second project, Alabama Agricultural Experiment Station researchers compared low-protein corn (7.7 percent) picked from plots receiving lower than optimum nitrogen with high-protein corn (11.0 to 12.5 percent) from soil receiving 3.5 times as much nitrogen.

To quote the publication, "The high-protein corn supported better growth of chicks and rats when equal amounts of corn were included in the diets.''

With plant protein declining—as some amino acids disappear—and carbohydrates increasing, strict vegetarian diets for weight loss become steadily more precarious for supporting life.

During a hearing before the Senate Select Committee on Nutrition and Human Needs, Allan Cott, M.D., observed that if all plants are to contain all trace minerals vital to supporting life, soils in which they grow must be given a complete fertilizer.[3]

However, for a century, many soils have been cultivated only with fertilizers composed of just nitrate, phosphate, potash, calcium, and magnesium. Consequently, many plant foods that we and animals eat are inadequate in trace elements.

Addressing the same committee, Michael Lesser, M.D., added a postscript. Government reports had revealed that the soil of thirty-two states was zinc-deficient and that commercial fertilizers return no zinc to the earth.[4]

On the other hand, copper plumbing has increased our intake of copper, upsetting our zinc-copper ratio, in which zinc must be dominant and in the right proportion.

Excess copper can trigger feelings of alienation, depression, and irritability, concluded Dr. Lesser.

Any of these symptoms can influence you to overeat.

One step removed from short-changed plants are processed foods, which represent another severe deduction in nutrients. Refined flour is a prime illustration of processing a product to death.

Several generations ago most whole grains were stone-ground, offering full food values. However, flour from such grain was harder to ship long distances without spoilage, so about a century ago, someone invented the high-speed roller mill, which separated the bran and germ, the nutritious parts, from the flour. These were fed to the hogs, and all the rest was reserved for human beings.

Our anemic flour ended up as anemic white bread, virtually innocent of nutrients. Twenty vitamins and minerals had been lost in processing. What once was the staff of life had become a broken crutch. Public pressure caused the so-called bread enrichment program, the addition of three vitamins and two minerals. If you subtract twenty nutrients and replace five, this is less an enrichment program than a decrease in impoverishment. Thanks to advertising double-talk, we are informed that enriched white bread is nourishing.

Further, chemicals added to age and bleach the flour destroy carotene, the vitamin A precursor, and what vitamin E remains, leaving amino acids and fats with chlorine residues.

Every vitamin and mineral deducted or destroyed, and every chemical added to white flour, is another reason for excluding bakery products made from them and soups and gravies thickened with them from your diet.

Also, sugar-laden breakfast foods, ideal for adding weight and developing dental caries, are noted for their snap, crackle, and pop. Just how nutritious can sound effects be?

Like packaged foods, canned products are permitted only

sparingly on the reducing diets of my patients because so many nutrients are lost to high temperatures in the canning process. One exception is canned salmon with its calcium-rich bones.

While fresh-frozen vegetables are preferable to canned varieties, they, too, have limitations. Their desperately needed trace minerals are often lost by chelating agents used in processing. Then, too, some salt or even sugar may be added to them.

For a host of reasons, including critical losses of nutrients in processing, foods in reducing diets are sure to shortchange you nutritionally because diet makers use nutrient values that are unrealistic.

It is customary to use raw food values deducted by 25 percent, supposedly to compensate for losses due to food storage, shipping, and exposure to light, oxygen, and elevated temperatures.

Inasmuch as 25 percent losses are far under the actual figure, you are taking in far fewer nutrients than you think on a reducing diet. Biochemist Richard Passwater notes that garden-fresh peas suffer a 56 percent loss of vitamins when cooked before serving.[5]

Frozen peas lose 83 percent in the process of scalding, freezing, thawing, and cooking. Canned peas sacrifice 94 percent of vitamins in scalding, sterilization, liquor diffusion, and reheating.

Enzymes decompose in fresh foods and cause rapid nutrient loss. Within several days, almost all the vitamin C migrates out of green vegetables. If you have a farm-fresh produce market nearby, buy your vegetables and fruits there, refrigerate them immediately to slow enzyme action, and use them quickly.

In canning, enzymatic action that would cause decomposition is stopped by scalding (bleaching). However, this protective measure also annihilates nutrients. (Many weight-loss diets include canned foods.)

Since your food may have been grown thousands of miles from your table, don't expect everything on your menu to have its estimated nutritional value.

While the revolution in food growing and distribution may

be a minor miracle in preventing starvation, it has marked short-comings nutritionally.

Eat most of your vegetables and fruit raw so that you don't lose valuable vitamins, minerals, and enzymes. If you must cook vegetables, do it with little water and at low heat. Of course, use the cooking liquid on the vegetables or in soup.

On the subject of enzymes, the clinical research of William H. Philpott, M.D.—cited in our book, *Solved: The Riddle of Illness*—reveals that an important cause of diabetes is eating too many processed foods devoid of enzymes. He claims that the pancreas cannot synthesize enough enzymes for the digestive process to make up for the dietary deficit.[6]

This is a major reason why I ask my patients to include at least one fresh fruit or vegetable with a meal.

On another subject, Willem H. Khoe, M.D., Ph.D., of Las Vegas, Nevada, cautions his patients about eating imitation foods: "If man made it, don't eat it."[7]

The major "don'ts" I mention to my patients are:

1. Don't eat imitation food products. (Real people need real food.)

2. Don't eat processed foods if you can get natural ones.

3. Don't eat canned foods if you can avoid them.

Let me elaborate about imitation foods. Why drink imitation milk, for example, when the real thing is in the same refrigerated area of your store? Why use artificial creamers on your cereals or in your hot beverages? If your object is to lower fat and cholesterol intake, remember that a main ingredient in many artificial creamers is coconut oil, one of the most saturated fats. Better use half and half, whole milk, or low or nonfat!

Any weight-loss diet should be rich in nutrients, not only vitamins and minerals but also enzymes, as well as low in calories. If it isn't, you risk losing your health and longevity along with pounds.

Not one of us needs that!

Some years ago, my collaborator Jim Scheer conducted an in-depth interview with the late Michael J. Walsh, Sc.D., F.R.I.C., one of the giants of biochemistry. In the early 1960s he pioneered personalized, scientifically computed dietary regimes.

Dr. Walsh made some startling revelations about why most dietary regimes are doomed to failure:

"Anyone with clinical experience in appraising food intakes of individuals, whether overweight or obese or of so-called ideal weight, is skeptical of the oversimplification that people are overweight because they overeat," he said.

Dr. Walsh, who wrote numerous articles for medical, dental, and nutritional journals, told of a survey he had made covering 4,500 cases referred to him by medical doctors and dentists.

Eighty-three percent of overweights were overweight while undereating—that is, on a diet lower than required for body maintenance. Only 17 percent were found to conform to the usually accepted belief that people are overweight because they overeat.

"Already the 83 percent were restricting calories and failing to lose weight. A common misconception holds that the human body should be viewed as parts of a whole on an additive-subtractive basis and if you weigh too much, you eat more than you need," stated Dr. Walsh.

"A more accurate basis of judgment is that the body consists of the sum of many organs and tissues, a dynamic, ever-changing organism as a whole in an ever-changing environment.

"What we are dealing with is function and consequence of altered and impaired function. The other popularly held basis is ingenuous and naive, a gross oversimplification of a highly complex subject," he stated.

"Relative to the 83 percent of cases associated with undereating, it makes much more sense to assume that overweight is a consequence of impaired metabolism, due to having eaten insufficient nutrient-appropriate food in the first place.

"Failing to get sufficient nutrients for body needs in order to survive, the organism slows down, lowering metabolism. An early consequence of lowered metabolism is retention of water in tissues, resulting in overweight, mistaken for fat.

"So what do you do for overweight or obesity? You act on the premise that reducing weight can be accomplished by eating foods which stimulate metabolism, the building of tissue, and the eliminating of superfluous water.

"In plainest terms, the more efficient way to lose weight —in the 83 percent of cases—is at the opposite pole from the conventional procedure. In order to lose weight, you eat more foods which are nutrient-rich. Instead of counting calories, you make each calorie count.

"Due to naive beliefs (often harmful) and misconceptions about calories and body weight held by most of the public (unfortunately, including many physicians and others connected with the health profession) many multiple vitamin mineral-protein deficiencies become routine. Therefore, you reap these consequences: (1) depleted tissues, (2) numerous unnecessary illnesses, and (3) a deranged metabolism resulting in overweight or obesity.

"No Fairy Godmother's magic wand will transform the insidious threats to our survival: soils which are steadily being depleted, a plain fact constantly varnished over by apologists; ingestion of too few nutrient-rich foods, and too many highly processed nutrient-poor foods.

"Refined cereals, breads, rolls, doughnuts, cookies, cakes, pies, hotcakes, waffles, syrups, and ice cream are labeled as good, delicious, refined or even natural foods, apparently supplying our every need for energy before our requirements for protein, minerals and vitamins are met.

"Such misuse of adjectives leads to inappropriate choices of foods, resulting in daily and, consequently, cumulative dietary deficiencies which cause metabolic imbalance and, therefore, lead to overweight," Dr. Walsh said.

Having followed the dietary history of several thousands of patients—not all overweight, of course—I am convinced of widely prevalent clinical and subclinical malnutrition. An upgrading of diet through judicious selection of foods with vitamin, mineral, and, often, enzyme supplementation not only improves health but enables the overweight and obese to lose—often with amazing ease.

Let's face the facts, the biochemical facts of life: Unless all required nutrients are included in your diet and/or supplements, fat cannot be efficiently burned.

If metabolism is reduced, you slow the rate at which fat burns and produces needed energy. Almost all nutrients you can name—and some you can't—are necessary for burning off fat, particularly the family of B vitamins. A lack of any B vitamin can reduce energy and heat and make you tired, if not exhausted. You will crave more food, usually refined carbohydrates.

Did you know that no matter how sincere your desire and how low your intake of refined carbohydrates or any group of foods, you will have difficulty ridding yourself of stored fat if your diet is deficient in vitamin B-6? When rats are slightly deficient of this nutrient, they burn fats and proteins so inefficiently that they become hopelessly obese.

Insufficient protein may also be a dietary hazard. If you short-change yourself of protein, you reduce the formation of energy-producing enzymes. Fat burns twice as fast—and, of course, more calories are used—when the diet is adequate in protein than when it is inadequate.

Also, insufficient vitamin E, processed out of most grains and flours, reduces fat utilization by one half, as has been shown by boosting the diet with this nutrient.

Some high-protein weight-loss diets either are ineffective or contribute to weight gain if deficient in vitamin B-6 and choline. Under this condition, protein rapidly turns to fat.

If your diet lacks lecithin, one of whose ingredients is choline, fat in your cells can't burn efficiently. This complicating factor also can lead to excess fats and cholesterol circulating in your blood and the possibility of high blood pressure, coronary artery disease, weight retention or gain, and fatigue or exhaustion.

Dietary deficiencies, especially vitamin B-2, pantothenic acid, and protein, combine with overweight to undermine liver function, reducing its ability to form enzymes needed to inactivate the hormone insulin. These shortages cause three devastating conditions to occur: super-high levels of insulin in the blood, the rapid formation of fats, and the equally rapid decline of blood sugar. As mentioned earlier, low blood sugar encourages weight gain and makes you always hungry.

In the light of facts presented, it is important to make calories count as well as to count calories.

18 | Melt Away Fat with Lo-Cal and No-Cal Diets

In earlier chapters, we observed that there is not just one kind of overweight or obesity. Therefore, one dietary approach may not work for all individuals. Cinderella's glass slipper won't fit everybody's foot, despite the fairy tales in many diet books.

As a respected international medical journal puts it, "No single diet exists for the treatment of obesity. On the contrary, a variety of diet regimes should be taken into consideration in this disease."[1]

Good advice.

You will have the chance to select the one right for you on the basis of comparative research. If you carry a heavy cargo of weight, you will also have the opportunity to consider fasting.

Which type of diet is more effective—the low- or high-carbohydrate? In a study not long ago, one group of obese test subjects was fed a low-carbohydrate diet and the other, a high-carbohydrate diet, both regimes equal at 1,000 kcal.[2]

The weight loss of individuals on the low-carbohydrate diet was significantly greater: a daily loss of 362 grams as opposed to 298 grams—approximately 18 percent greater.

Then the intake of both diets was raised to 1,900 kcal daily. Again, the mean weight loss on the low-carbohydrate diet was significantly greater than on the high-carbohydrate diet: 351 grams per day versus 296 grams per day—again approximately 18 percent greater for the former.

In biochemical circles, heated argument still arises as to whether to accent carbohydrates or protein in low-calorie diets. Eleven considerably overweight healthy young women were subjected to one of two very low-calorie regimes: 360 Kcal in Diet A (all protein) and 340 kcal in Diet B (all carbohydrates).[3] After three weeks, researchers found no significant difference in weight or in seven biochemical measurements.

Another much debated question is whether fats or carbohydrates raise the metabolism higher, generate more body heat, and utilize more calories in the process. Research reported in *Metabolism* compared the heat response in a high-fat meal and a high-carbohydrate meal in normal-weight and obese subjects.[4]

The metabolic rate of test subjects was measured before and for six hours after a meal. Blood samples were taken every thirty minutes to measure insulin, blood sugar, and catecholamines.

The high-fat meal produced less heat than the high-carbohydrate meal. The study's most telltale finding was that normal-weight subjects generated more heat than the obese patients and, therefore, tended to retain little, if any, fat.

HEAVYWEIGHTS ARE CARBOHYDRATE PRONE

And, speaking of carbohydrates, is it true that overweight persons prefer carbohydrates above other food groups? Possibly.

Two respected authorities, J. J. Wurtman and P. J. Wurtman, have observed that almost all excess eating by the obese can be accounted for by carbohydrate snacks. However, their research with obese human beings reveals that carbohydrate craving is not necessarily governed only by taste of carbohydrates or the need for calories. They suggest that brain mechanisms independent of these two considerations cause the craving.[5]

One of the Wurtmans' experiments revealed that d-fenfluramine, a serotonin-releasing drug, reduces the desire of obese individuals to eat the carbohydrates that put on excess weight. However, it does not diminish the tendency for them to eat proteins.

DON'T NEGLECT YOUR TRYPTOPHAN!

Since I practice treating patients as much as possible without drugs, I have my carbohydrate cravers take at least 667 mg of tryptophan daily. Tryptophan, an essential amino acid—it cannot be synthesized by the human body—is necessary for the formation of serotonin. This amino acid is particularly effective when taken with a small amount of carbohydrate and with a low-protein meal.

Tryptophan is especially important to those who want to lose because it encourages sound sleep. Disordered sleep and long periods of wakefulness give the overweight more chance to think about food, to crave it, and to be tempted to raid the refrigerator.

The best natural food sources of tryptophan are chicken, cheddar cheese, milk, tuna, turkey, soybeans, and products derived from the latter: tofu, for example.

Don't overlook the value of tryptophan-rich foods and/or tryptophan supplement in curbing your appetite for carbohydrates. One of a number of surveys shows that overweight individuals are drawn to refined carbohydrates and fats: potato chips, corn snacks, pretzels, crackers, cookies, doughnuts, sweet rolls, cake, and candy, as well as frozen dairy desserts and fresh and processed meat. Many of the latter are loaded with sodium, which encourages fluid retention.[6]

Commenting in *The International Journal of Obesity* on today's carbohydrate craze, British weight-control authority P. J. Bradley calls the modern trend toward overweight "not simply a metabolic or behavioral disorder." Rather, it is based on an "evolutionary adaptation to modern food, particularly the refined carbohydrates."[7]

The provocative Bradley statement has much validity. Certainly, diminishing the intake of refined carbohydrates would help in the weight control of many individuals. However, it is just a single, important approach to a complex problem which has many answers.

DOES FASTING PAY OFF?

In this vein, some weight-control specialists believe in extreme measures, particularly in the grossly obese. One of the most extreme, aside from surgery, is fasting. Other authorities do not favor the long fast; on the rebound, patients often return to their old eating habits with a vengeance, quickly taking on all the padding they had lost if not more.

In addition, fasting has its hazards. Patients have been known to die during a fast or, at least, to suffer severe malnourishment with an accent on neuropathies, deterioration of nerves that may cause a limitation of arm, leg, or eye function. However, the latter often can be prevented by a daily intake of at least 50 mg of vitamin B-complex. Sometimes iodine is also deficient, and hypothyroidism contributes to neuropathies, too. If iodine fails to help, supplementation with natural thyroid hormone often can.

Still other common deficiencies among fasters are minerals: calcium, magnesium, potassium, and phosphorus, with consequent deterioration of bones (not always immediately detectable), teeth, and the substructures of teeth. Bones and teeth are the calcium banks whose accounts are frequently overdrawn to keep the blood supplied with this mineral.

Then, too, fasting reduces sexuality in men, and encourages menstrual problems in women. It contributes to adrenal exhaustion, gout, and stomach ulcers in both sexes.

Despite the hazards of fasting, I have prescribed it for a small number of obese or extremely overweight patients, but always under close supervision. One cannot be too careful, especially in long-term fasting.

MERITS OF THE MODIFIED FAST

I prefer to use modified fasting along the lines of Swedish doctors who prescribe fresh vegetable and fruit juices: at least a quart of juices daily, diluted with an equal amount of water, a base for vitamin and mineral supplements.[8] Carrot juice is my patients' favorite vegetable juice, and fresh apple the favorite fruit juice. I sometimes permit orange or grapefruit juice for patients who are not allergic to them.

Here are the Mega Weight Loss System's vitamins and minerals for my heavyset patients on a modified fast:

Vitamin A	10,000 I.U. (derived from fish liver oil).
Vitamin B-complex:	50 mg of major fractions.
Vitamin C:	4,000 mg.
Vitamin E:	400 I.U. (alpha tocoperol).
Calcium (oyster shell with 400 I.U. vitamin D):	1,000 mg.
Magnesium	500 mg.
Potassium	550 mg.
Selenium	50 mcg.
Tryptophan	667 mg.
Zinc	25 mg.

On a modified fast, my patients come out in better health than those on a total fast, and, over two to four weeks, lose an average of twelve to twenty-four pounds. This is comparable with losses reported by Swedish doctors using a similar regime but without vitamin-mineral supplementation.

Further, as with patients of the Swedish doctors, the heavy-weights lowered their cholesterol, gained a more favorable ratio of high-density lipoproteins (HDL) to low-density lipoproteins (LDL), and also reduced their triglyceride levels.

Some of my colleagues report successful weight loss of thirty or more pounds by their patients due to fasting for thirty to forty days without serious or permanent deterioration of health. But, of course, this is not for diabetics or those suffering from heart or kidney disease.

Total fasting does work, despite its negative aspects, but I only recommend it if obesity is seriously impairing the health or life of a patient.

A study of 207 obese persons hospitalized to achieve significant weight loss through uninterrupted fasting revealed that 79 patients succeeded in reducing to 30 percent of their ideal weight.[9]

Most of the test subjects maintained their weight reduction for at least a year and a half, no matter how much poundage they had lost. After two to three years, half of the patients had regained their original obesity, and nine years later, fewer than 10 percent were able to remain lighter than when they had started fasting.

DO FASTERS FIND FASTING WORTHWHILE?

Despite this sad reversion, most patients found the fasting experience well worthwhile. The temporary weight loss brought them a higher quality of life and improved health as well as other benefits: far more employment opportunities (including greater social acceptance) and higher earnings.

Test subjects also derived psychological bonuses: a feeling of control over their fat, the feeling that the abrupt change would break the grip of previous dietary habits, and encouragement that significant weight loss was possible for them after all.

Is it difficult to fast?

Yes, for the first week. After that, the intense craving for food decreases and makes fasting easily tolerable.

The fact that only 10 percent of the 207 obese subjects mentioned earlier were able to maintain weight less than at the start of the study indicates a profound truth: fasting may offer benefits, but none of us can live forever without food. Therefore, it makes the most sense to establish a realistic weight-loss goal, modify your diet, and change your way of life to support a leaner, happier YOU.

Above all, a reducing diet must be practical, appeal to the senses, and provide fewer calories than energy expended—or you will soon scuttle it.

Dr. Leslie Sandlow, quoted earlier, points out a flaw in most weight-loss diets. They are doomed to failure unless planned with *you* in mind, rather than some nameless, faceless, average person. They must have some of the foods that you like. (All of them are not necessarily allergens and addictive.)

While urging a balanced diet, Dr. Sandlow advises: "Don't deprive yourself of what you crave, or your diet will seem like torture, and you'll quit."

Grant Gwinup, M.D., professor and chairman of Endocrinology and Metabolism, University of California, Irvine, has found that drastic dietary changes from your customary ratio of protein, carbohydrate, and fat are usually impractical and self-defeating. [10]

"Extreme changes make it difficult to stay on the new diet. You still have the old food cravings and soon will be back on your former regime."

Dr. Gwinup leans toward learning to live with a little hunger, because when you are hungry, you start to burn off fat.

Another school of thought favors a proper orchestration of carbohydrates, proteins, and fats to keep you satiated so you won't be hungry and overeat. Carbohydrates leave the stomach fastest; proteins linger there longer and fats stay the longest, often three or four hours. Therefore, if you sharply reduce fat in your diet, hunger will assail you earlier.

Fiber, too, delays the onset of hunger pangs but by means of another physiological process. Its bulk gives you a feeling of fullness for a long period. For this and other reasons fiber is a *must* for the weight-loss diet of most individuals, especially those who have been eating mainly processed foods.

However, the contributions of fiber, an important component in the Mega Weight Loss Diet, are too major to be confined to a few paragraphs.

Fiber deserves a chapter all its own.

19 | Fiber—The Fabulous Food

A few chapters ago, we mentioned the valuable parts of the wheat grain removed by processing. One of them, bran, has been made part of the F-Plan Diet, a weight-control regime featuring fiber.

Called roughage in grandma's day, fiber hurries food through your digestive system, slows down the absorption of carbohydrates, and delays the sensation of hunger.

Much documentation shows that fiber does help dieters lose weight. But it has limitations, as will be explained later.

Too many of us tend to think of fiber as just wheat bran. It is that and more. Although wheat bran is the richest source of fiber per one-third cup—6.4 grams—there are other excellent fibrous foods: oat bran, 4.2 grams; brown rice, approximately 2.00 grams; and wheat germ, 1.8, among the grains; kidney beans, 5 grams; navy beans, 4.3; split peas, 4.3; white beans, 4.2; lima beans, 4.0; blackberries, 4.00 per half cup; dried prunes (three large) 3.7; apples, approximately 2.1 with skin.

HOW MUCH YOU NEED

Various surveys indicate that the average daily diet contains only about 15 grams of fiber, approximately half of the 25 to 30 grams recommended by the National Cancer Institute.

Although some nutritionists praise fiber's contributions to good health, others remind us that, in reducing the number of calories absorbed, fiber also reduces the amount of nutrients absorbed.

Some authorities even warn us away from a super-high-fiber weight-reduction diet that includes all the whole grains, legumes, fruits, and vegetables you can eat. Such a diet could be too much of a good thing, warns Judith Levine, San Francisco registered dietician for the American Heart Association and the Dairy Council of California.

Fiber is a must, she admits, but a diet should not exclude essential nutrients such as protein, calcium, and iron found in dairy products and in various meats.

Large amounts of bran added to foods can cause dehydration and digestive tract ailments, she states. Therefore, fiber should be added to the diet gradually and should be accompanied by plenty of fluids: at least eight to ten glasses daily.

If used in excess, wheat and oat bran can cause nutritional deficiencies.[1] Their phytic acid attaches itself to calcium, copper, iron, magnesium, and zinc and strong-arms considerable amounts of these essential minerals out of the body. The harm of mineral deficiencies is best illustrated by poor teeth and various kinds of bone degeneration in relation to insufficient calcium.

MANY BENEFITS

On the positive side, much evidence indicates that fiber contributes greatly to our good health. A publication in *Postgraduate Medicine Journal* suggests that intake of cereal fiber (not bran) prevents secondary bile salt recycling from the colon and contributing to overproduction of cholesterol. So far as encouraging weight loss is concerned, the writer of this publication states that long-term intake of such fiber is as important as a low-fat diet.[2]

Several studies show that fiber reduces cholesterol levels and, in many instances, brings about a more favorable ratio of high-density lipoproteins (HDL) to low-density lipoproteins (LDL). Fiber also lowers the blood level of other fats. Fiber gives us double service in reducing cholesterol and, therefore, lessens the stress of concern about it.

Fiber has an exciting track record for helping hearts to remain healthy. Not long ago *Lancet* reported dramatic results of a 10-year study of 871 middle-aged men in Zutphen, Netherlands. Test subjects who ate 27 grams or less of fiber daily (roughly an ounce) had a heart attack death rate four times greater than persons who took in 37 grams or more.[3]

Another report indicates that unprocessed wheat bran "significantly reduced blood sugar and plasma immunoreactive insulin concentration on the glucose tolerance test of obese children." For this reason, the authors found that obese children can benefit in many ways from a supplement of unprocessed bran.[4]

Still another study concludes that in obesity and other metabolic disorders, it is a good idea to include low-calorie foods high in fiber along with low-fat foods such as soy dishes, pectin-enriched dishes, fruit purees, skimmed milk and yogurt, along with wheat-bran biscuits.[5]

LOADED WITH NUTRIENTS

So heavy an accent is put on the fact that wheat bran is super-high in fiber that many of us think of it as containing *nothing* nutritional. On the contrary, wheat bran is a *super* food, rich in protein, B-vitamins, and in minerals. A half cup of wheat bran —about 100 grams—boasts 80 percent as much protein as a serving of meat and liberal amounts of the following B vitamins: .72 mg of B-1 (only brewer's yeast and wheat germ have a higher content); .35 mg of B-2 (just milk, liver, and yeast have more of this vitamin); 21 mg of niacin (only yeast has a higher content of this vitamin); 2.9 mg of pantothenic acid (liver alone is richer in this vitamin); .82 of B-6 (only liver and sunflower seeds have higher amounts).

As for minerals, bran has 1,121 mg of phosphorus and an equal amount of potassium (higher than all foods but brewer's yeast); 14.9 mg of iron (only brewer's yeast and wheat germ are richer in content); and 490 mg of magnesium (no other foods can boast this high a content).[6]

Of course, such nutritional bonuses are especially important in low-calorie weight-control diets, but we look to bran as well as other fiber-rich foods—fresh vegetables, fruit, legumes, nuts, and seeds—mainly for the physiological benefits contributed by their fiber.

First, there are an estimated 150 to 250 different types of fiber, most of them found in foods, but only two major categories: indigestible, the type found in grains, bran of wheat, corn, oats, or rice and the digestible, mucilagelike kinds in seeds and gum-rich foods—alginates, carageenan, guar gum, agar-agar, and pectin.

DIFFERENT STROKES

Although all types of fiber make similar contributions to our health and weight, they don't all make equal contributions.

Fiber from corn, oats, or wheat bran is best for prevention of constipation, gastrointestinal disorders, diverticulosis, and colon cancer. However, pectin and guar are more effective in keeping our after-meals blood sugar normal. Again, our major interest is weight control.

Great Britain's Denis Burkitt, M.D., deserves plaudits for his revealing research that showed the numerous benefits of fiber. I learned from him that five slices of whole-*meal* bread—not whole wheat—increased bowel weight as much as seven-plus pounds of apples.

How can fiber work its weight-loss wonders? First, it has few or no calories and offers much bowel bulk because of its spongelike ability to take on water—as much as eight or nine times its dry weight. It makes you feel full and less likely to overeat.

It takes longer to eat fibrous food. A heavy slice of whole-grain bread demands chewing, unlike the limp, doughy white bread. Chewing stimulates the production of digestive juices in your mouth.

An experiment by the U.S. Department of Agriculture and the University of Maryland showed less efficient digestibility of high fiber foods—a decrease of 4.8 percent in digestibility of calories. This means that almost 5 percent of the calories passed through instead of staying in the body.

This was proved by twelve men who lived on a low-fiber diet for twenty-six days and then switched to a high-fiber one—fresh fruits and vegetables (no whole grains).

More pertinent to weight loss is the fact that some fibers—especially guar gum and soy fiber—slow the uptake of sugar in the small intestine, helpful in the treatment of diabetes.

HELPS IN DIABETES AND WEIGHT LOSS

Such evidence has been developed by studies of Dr. James Anderson, chief of endocrinology at the University of Kentucky Medical Center, who recommends dietary control of diabetes with 25 grams of fiber daily and a diet consisting of 70 percent complex carbohydrates (with 10 percent natural sugar), 15 percent protein, and 15 percent fat.[7]

Fiber has a profound effect on how the body's energy-use system responds to the intake of sugar. One experiment compared blood-sugar response of test subjects to a sugary liquid and to the same liquid with the addition of a form of fibers: pectin.[8]

In the first instance, blood sugar shot upward. In the second it remained near normal. Fiber had kept blood sugar from an abnormal rise and, at the same time, had sharply reduced the insulin response by 50 percent.

Still more evidence shows the value of fiber in influencing the energy-use system. Pectin-free apple juice sent blood insulin levels of test subjects 50 percent higher than those others who ingested an equal number of calories in whole apples.

Fiber's stabilizing influence prevents the sharp rise and consequent devastating decline in blood glucose, which makes for the hypoglycemic's constant hunger accompanied by emotional symptoms such as depression, still another stimulant for over-eating.

BONUS VALUES

In addition, fiber provides an ideal environment for friendly intestinal bacteria. It absorbs poisonous heavy metals—mercury and lead—and draws them out of the body. Fibrous food also discourages tooth decay by removing dental plaque during the chewing process, and by replacing soft carbohydrates such as white bread that adhere to the teeth.

Fiber seems to help prevent obesity and diabetes in individuals who tend toward them genetically. It is protective in both instances.

Such upbeat reports about fiber encourage individuals to eat fiber in inordinate amounts. Initially, this often is a shock to the system, particularly when fluid intake has not been increased. If a person tends to be constipated, additional fiber without additional fluids can intensify constipation.

MAKE HASTE SLOWLY

The best advice I can give about using fiber is to proceed with caution. Start with a teaspoon a day of bran on your morning oatmeal, wheat, rye, or millet cereal, and just add a glass of water to your normal fluid intake. After a week, add another teaspoon and a little more fluid.

Too much fiber too soon can cause intestinal distress, or diarrhea and flatulence. An over-zealous patient of mine disregarded this precaution and suffered more inflation than a nation with a rampant economy.

A comprehensive study reported in the *British Journal of Nutrition* gave one special fiber extremely high grades for effectiveness: guar gum, which is available in many drug stores and in most nutrition centers.[9]

ONE-MAN ARMY IN THE WEIGHT WAR

Guar gum came out of experiments looking like a one-product army to win the war against overweight. First, it reduced hunger "significantly better than commercially available bran taken in the same way," based on hunger ratings recorded daily for ten weeks. Second, it raised the metabolism of carbohydrates and fats, a big advantage for the overweight and the obese. Third, guar gum reduced blood sugar after meals. A single dose reduced blood glucose levels by 10 percent. Blood insulin levels were essentially unchanged, suggesting that cell responsiveness to insulin was increased.

An additional benefit to test subjects was significant reduction of blood cholesterol with long-term usage. However, high-density lipoproteins remained unchanged.

The most encouraging result of this experiment was that body weight of obese subjects was significantly reduced by guar gum intake, although patients were asked to stay on their usual diets—a remarkable result.

Guar gum comes with glowing letters of reference based on impressive testing.

Now other New Age nutrients are invading nutrition centers, drug stores, and supermarkets with the purpose of helping you lose weight and keep it lost.

You may want to consider some of them in the next chapter.

20 | New Age Nutrients and the Bathroom Scale

Speaking of fiber for weight-control, much heralded glucomannan, considered a New Age nutrient in the English-speaking world, is anything but a Johnny-come-lately.

For almost 1,000 years, the konjac plant from whose root it is derived has been a food and promoter of regularity in Japan.

Today, glucomannan is beginning to win recognition for its ability to decrease appetite and help dieters to stay on a low-calorie regime. Some of my obese patients have tried it and have done quite well.

Glucomannan, a granular product, is ingested before a meal in a glass of water and swells by eight to nine times its dry volume. It makes you feel so full that you can easily resist over-eating.

Although many members of the medical profession are skeptical about the merits of glucomannan, there is some documentation that validates its effectiveness in a weight-loss program.

FAVORABLE RESULTS

An eight-week double-blind study reported in the *International Journal of Obesity* revealed that glucomannan definitely contributes to weight loss.[1]

Twenty obese test subjects took two 500 mg capsules of glucomannan or a look-alike placebo with an eight ounce glass of water one hour before three meals each day. All participants were told not to change either their usual eating or exercise habits.

Those who took the glucomannan lost 5.5 pounds over eight weeks. Furthermore, both their serum cholesterol and low-density lipoprotein, LDL, the "Bad Guy" cholesterol, were reduced by 21.7 and 15.0 mg/dl, respectively. None of this happened with the placebo takers. No adverse reactions were reported in the glucomannan group.

However, this food supplement, like other fibers, can remove valuable nutrients along with calories. As a countermeasure, I recommend that glucomannan be taken before only two meals a day and skipped before the most nourishing meal, the one with which most of the day's food supplements are taken.

This helps correct the problem. The individuals lose poundage somewhat more slowly, but they also lose fewer nutrients. They realize the best of both worlds.

Two other New Age nutrients that show great promise in weight reduction are carnitine and gamma-linolenic acid (GLA).

CARNITINE ACCELERATES FAT BURNING

Carnitine, also called vitamin B_T, speeds the burning of fat. When the body shows a high level of carnitine, body fat burns at a high rate. Just the opposite is true when levels of this nutrient are low.

Researchers I. B. Fritz, of the University of Michigan, and K. T. N. Yue, spent many years trying to determine how carnitine accelerates fat burning in the cells. Finally they discovered the secret.[2]

They found that the cells' mitochondria, mini-furnaces or powerplants where fats and carbohydrates are translated into energy, were impenetrable by fats. It turned out that carnitine, with help from an enzyme at the inner mitochondria wall, links with fat and transports it into the mitochondria for burning. A low supply of carnitine, then, could slow down the delivery process and leave surplus fat to accumulate.

Can the body synthesize carnitine, or must it be taken in through food or food supplements?

The answer to this two-headed question is that the body can, indeed, synthesize carnitine, but of course it cannot do so without proper nutritional raw materials.

Diets deficient in the amino acids lysine and methionine and vitamin C, as well as carnitine itself, seem to slow down or shut down the carnitine-synthesizing mechanism.

The richest food sources of carnitine are muscle meats of sheep, lamb, beef, and chicken. Although all foods have not been analyzed to determine carnitine content, it has been found that yeast, milk, and wheat germ contain appreciable amounts.

NOT IN VEGETABLES AND FRUIT

Vegetables and fruit contain only negligible amounts of carnitine, so vegetarians do not have the benefit of this nutrient. Further, vegetarian regimes are usually low in lysine and methionine, amino acids that must be present for carnitine synthesis to take place in the body.

Two studies, one by the prestigious Mayo Clinic, have established that we make four times as much carnitine as we take in by diet.[3]

Several categories of individuals have been found to be low in blood and tissue levels of carnitine: those on a fast, the hospitalized on intravenous nutrition, dialysis patients, strenuous exercisers over prolonged periods, and the obese.

In an earlier chapter, we mentioned that thyroid hormones act as a carburetor to govern call metabolism. The same thing might be said for carnitine, relative to fat burning in cells. That is why this nutrient may be an important food supplement for losing weight.

SIGNIFICANT FINDING

An experiment by researchers at the American McGaw firm demonstrates this point. Test animals were induced to develop fatty livers. Then they were fed carnitine supplements, and soon the liver fat began to dissipate. How quickly the fat disappeared was in direct proportion to how much their carnitine intake was increased.[4]

A number of human studies have also shown that carnitine can help reduce fat-storage areas in various parts of the body.

Research at the University of British Columbia revealed that mice that were genetically prone to be obese had almost 50 percent less carnitine than mice genetically prone to stay lean.[5]

It seems that this nutrient has a bright future in weight reduction. However, more research, including double-blind studies, would help to fill numerous knowledge gaps.

Carnitine, the safety of which has been said to be established, is available in nutrition centers and in some drug stores. The experience of my patients with carnitine has not yet been conclusive. I can only say that it appears to work best with a reduced-calorie regime and a vigorous exercise program.

Another promising food supplement for stimulating weight loss is gamma-linolenic acid (GLA). There is considerable research that validates its value for this purpose. Therefore, you will find it among the key supplements to my Mega Weight Loss Diet in the next chapter.

EVENING PRIMROSE OIL GLA: A BIG HELP

Various experiments show that GLA blocks the laying down of fat deposits in four ways: (1) by reducing appetite; (2) by activating one of the body's greatest energy users, enzyme systems that keep potassium and sodium in proper ratio in each of our trillions of cells; (3) by triggering the operation of brown fat; and (4) by inhibiting the making of fat from carbohydrates.[6]

GLA is a rare substance—so rare that it is found plentifully only in mother's milk and in evening primrose oil, derived from seeds of the evening primrose plant whose flowers bloom on only one night of the year. Approximately 8 to 9 percent of evening primrose oil is GLA.

Thanks to Agricultural Seed Holdings Ltd., a British seed

company, a steady supply of the richest evening primrose oil was developed. This company conducted an extensive search, located 1,000 varieties of the evening primrose, selected the best quality, and developed plants with the most abundant yield of highest quality oil.

ACCIDENTAL DISCOVERY

Two researchers independently, accidentally, and simultaneously discovered the weight-loss-encouraging potential of Evening Primrose Oil (*Efamol*): David Horrobin, Ph.D., in Canada, and Dr. K. S. Vaddadi in England. Checking the use of this oil for possible side effects, Dr. Horrobin enlisted normal test subjects, some of whom were overweight. Half of the latter lost weight with no attempt to diet. Some even found that their appetites were reduced.[7]

While administering evening primrose oil to psychiatric patients, Dr. Vaddadi observed that nurses were taking capsules of this substance because they had seen that overweight patients were losing weight.

Learning of each other's findings, the two doctors jointly reported their research results, one of which was that normal-weight individuals showed no weight change while taking it, but that half of the overweights on it lost significant poundage without dieting.

WHEN THE SCALE IS STUCK

One particular experiment shows the special niche for evening primrose oil in weight loss. In the Metabolic Unit at the University of Wales, ten extremely obese subjects—40 percent above ideal weight—had stopped reducing on a 1,000-calorie diet. Then they were given six evening primrose oil capsules each day along with their diet, and they started losing again: 4.8 Kg (roughly ten and one-half pounds) at the end of six weeks.[8]

Further, sodium content in red blood cells fell significantly, showing that the evening primrose oil had activated this high-energy burning enzyme system in cells throughout the body. Some of these patients also had their brown fat activity monitored by thermography, which revealed that the evening primrose oil had dramatically expanded the active brown fat area, a phenomenon that the diet only regime of other test subjects did not accomplish.

Experiments with genetically obese mice showed that evening primrose oil limited weight gain compared with control animals, suggesting that this product may be effective in the specific problem areas of the obese: fundamental flaws in metabolism. In such cases, evening primrose oil can limit weight gain and cause weight loss.

Relative to these experiments, Dr. Horrobin hastens to point out that evening primrose oil is not likely to work when obesity results from overeating only.

His findings lead to the rationale for my weight loss program, which limits daily food intake to 1,000 calories and includes, among its supplements, two 500 mg capsules of Evening Primrose Oil (*Efamol*) three times a day.*

The last chapter of this book deals with the Mega Weight Loss Diet. It explains how it differs from any other diet ever offered and why it is effective.

---

* Available from Nature's Way Products, Inc., 10 Mountain Springs Parkway, Springville, Utah, 84663, 1-800-962-8873.

21 | Mega Weight Loss Diet
or
Chop Suey for *Breakfast?*

I remember reading a column by the *New York Times* syndicate's Jane Brody, who mentioned enjoying dinner leftovers for breakfast.

This is indeed a sensible idea for two reasons: (1) We forego a lot of excellent foods by staying in the typical breakfast rut of juice, eggs, toast, and coffee, and furthermore, (2) leftovers should be eaten quickly to minimize oxidation, exposure to light, and possible yeast growth, as mentioned by Dr. Crook in the chapter *The Yeast Crisis and Overweight*.

Speaking of the breakfast rut, one of my patients took a lot of good-natured needling for mentioning having eaten leftover chop suey for breakfast.

I encouraged him, so long as the chop suey contained no monosodium glutamate.

To make the Mega Weight Loss Diet work, you may have to become more adaptable in the kinds of foods you eat, particularly for breakfast. I'm not talking about a single food or even a single food group. As already mentioned, this is folly and could even help you gain weight. I mean being unconventional in not insisting that certain foods must be eaten at certain meals.

It may make more sense to eat chop suey for breakfast—the heavy meal to give yourself energy for the day—rather than for dinner, when you may need little energy (as covered in detail in the chapter *Three Squares Could Make you Round*).

A not-so-unconventional aspect of this diet is that it lessens the amount of fat in or on frequently eaten foods.

Some studies indicate that excess ingestion of fat contributes to added poundage. Barbara Bassett, editor/publisher of *Bestways*, a leading health and nutrition magazine, has certain favorite ways of reducing fat in the diet.

You may already be using some of her strategies and could benefit by using all of them:

1. Slicing visible fat from meat and poultry.

2. Removing skin from poultry before baking or roasting.

3. Cooking soups and stews a day earlier than needed, so you can skim off congealed fat before reheating.

4. Browning food in nonstick pans to eliminate cooking fats.

5. Using plain, low-, or nonfat yogurt in place of sour cream on baked potatoes. Yogurt can be blended with mayonnaise to reduce fat and calories and, also, to add to finished sauces.

6. Ordering salad dressings and sauces on the side in restaurants. This is one way you can control quantities used.

7. Serving finger food vegetables—carrot, celery, green pepper sticks, and radishes—rather than dressed salads.

8. Using nonstick spray coating, preferably containing lecithin, instead of greasing or buttering baking pans or casseroles.

9. Using low-fat, low-calorie mayonnaise and salad dressings in place of the others.

10. Eating nuts more often than nut butters. The former contain roughly 50 calories per tablespoon. The latter have about twice that much.

It will be understood that you take these measures—particularly slicing fat off meat and removing skin from poultry—in connection with the weight loss program as a whole.

The Mega Weight Loss Diet is unique in having been designed to consider all relevant factors in earlier chapters—not merely caloric input as opposed to caloric output (typical of the usual diet), but hypothyroidism, Candida albicans (a variation on the basic regime), hypoglycemia, food sensitivities and allergies, stress, heavy metals intoxication, and the immune system. Its specal features are:

1. The heaviest meal in the morning, a lighter one at noon, and the lightest one at night, with mid-morning and mid-afternoon snacks.

2. Daily intake of calories spread over five feedings, increasing the possibility of greater weight loss and assuring stable blood sugar to rule out emotional states such as depression, which encourage overeating. (See Chapter 4, *Killing Me Sweetly*.)

3. Rotation of foods on a five-day basis in the Dr. Max Rinkel tradition for the purpose of eliminating or at least minimizing food sensitivities and allergies, as covered in Chapter 5, *Lose Allergies and Weight*.

4. Eating a fresh vegetable or fruit—none of the latter on the Candida albicans diet—with each major meal to supply enzymes, most of which are lost in processed foods. (Enzymes are essential to digesting food, extracting its nutrients, and incorporating them into our trillions of cells. They are often overlooked in most weight-loss diets.)

5. Sufficient fiber to promote regularity and good health, to help rid the body of heavy metals, to stabilize blood sugar, and, of course, to encourage weight loss.

6. Simple menus for two reasons: (1) to minimize chances of food sensitivities and allergies common to multi-ingredient dishes—the fewer the ingredients, the better—and (2) to make food preparation easy enough to overcome resistance to cooking.

7. Food supplements to compensate for the near impossibility of getting sufficient nutrients in so few calories. (In my nutrition-oriented practice and in my capacity as president of the American Nutritional Medical Association, I have found that few diets—high- or low-calorie—do much more than sustain life, sometimes

poorly, at that. Real living means being healthy, vigorous, and zestful.)

Before offering you the Mega Weight Loss Diet, let me draw the zipper closed on this book by offering several recommendations.

First, give yourself every opportunity to lose the weight you wish by ruling out hypothyroidism, Candida albicans, hypoglycemia, food sensitivities and allergies, severe stress, heavy metals intoxication, and a weakened immune system. If you have one or more of them, seek successful treatment.

Remember, before you can lose weight permanently, you must eliminate these common, often subtle, usually undetected causes for overweight.

Then set a realistic weight-loss goal and a reasonable time to reach it. A pound a week is realistic for most of my patients.

Use the various motivations offered earlier, including the Davis system for developing sustained motivation, for changing won't power to willpower.

Review Chapter 12 to recall how to develop new habit patterns.

Try the Grant Gwinup regime of thirty or more minutes a day of aerobic exercises to rev up your heat-generating, fat-burning systems—that is, once your doctor okays it. Remember that the women in Dr. Gwinup's experiment didn't start losing weight steadily until they reached the thirty-or-more-minute level of daily aerobic workouts.

The Mega Weight Loss Diet will offer you a pattern for more small meals daily, with the accent on the heaviest meal in the morning. Follow it.

Forget about shortcuts to spectacular weight loss. They don't and won't work. Try the long, steady way. It will pay.

My first inclination is to wish you luck. However, if you follow the entire program, you are going to lose the desired amount of weight, and you won't need good luck.

You can do it. I *know* you can!

Following are two Mega Weight Loss Diets: the basic 1,000 calorie daily regime and the second one for individuals who have Candida albicans, also 1,000 calories.

In each instance, the diet is followed by a list of food supplements to be taken, too. The diet and the supplements are a team. Don't break up the team.

The ball is in your court!

DR. LANGER'S MEGA WEIGHT LOSS DIET
Approximately 1,000 calories

BASIC DIET
Five-Day Rotation

(List of supplements to be taken daily with food follows the Fifth Day of this diet.)

FIRST DAY

Breakfast

Lean ground meat or white meat chicken or turkey, baked or
    broiled, 4 oz
Carrot, crunchy or grated
Milk, 2 percent fat

Mid-Morning Snack

Muffin, buckwheat or bran

Lunch

Eggs, two, medium, soft or hardboiled
Green salad, Romaine lettuce, all you can eat, with safflower oil
    dressing and a hint of iodized sea salt
Coffee substitute, freshly brewed

Mid-Afternoon Snack

Sunflower seeds, unsalted, 1 oz

Dinner

Yam, medium size, baked (lower in calories than a sweet potato)
Cabbage-carrot salad, grated, unsweetened yogurt dressing
Chamomile tea

SECOND DAY

Breakfast

Oatmeal with soy milk
Toast, whole grain rye, lightly buttered
Orange, Valencia, medium size
Coffee substitute, freshly brewed

Mid-Morning Snack

Popcorn, air-popped and lightly buttered, 1 cup

Lunch

Lentil soup
Green salad: Romaine lettuce, alfalfa sprouts, olive oil dressing
Watermelon, ½ slice of 10″ × 1″ round
Spring water

Mid-Afternoon Snack

Cauliflower florets, 4

Dinner

Irish potato, small, baked in skin, lightly buttered, sprinkled with
    dill and iodized sea salt
Green pepper strips, six
Strawberries, fresh, 16 medium or 8 large
Spring water

THIRD DAY

Breakfast

Millet, cooked, one pat of butter
Pear, fresh
Coffee substitute, freshly brewed

Mid-Morning Snack

Pumpkin seeds, unsalted, 1 oz

Lunch

Salmon patty blended with freshly diced onion, broiled, 3 oz
Jicama slices, three
Spring water

Mid-Afternoon Snack

Celery stalk, small, with almond butter

Dinner

Green salad, butter lettuce, all you can eat, with soy dressing,
    hint of iodized sea salt
Sweet corn, small ear, lightly buttered and seasoned with iodized
    sea salt
Apricots, fresh, two
Spring water

FOURTH DAY

Breakfast

Veal chop, broiled, 3 oz
Muffin, oat bran
Cantaloupe, cubed, one cup
Coffee substitute, freshly brewed or herb tea

Mid-Morning Snack

Almonds, unsalted, 7

Lunch

Tuna salad with Boston lettuce (3 oz tuna) with sunflower seed
    oil dressing with a touch of iodized sea salt
Tangerine, medium
Herb tea

Mid-Afternoon Snack

Pecans, 10 large halves

Dinner

Brown rice, short grain, ½ cup cooked and flavored with beef
    broth
Red raspberries, fresh, unsweetened, ½ cup
Spring water

FIFTH DAY

You have the option of going back to the First Day or of using this, then following through the cycle from the Second Day through the Fourth Day.

Breakfast

Omelet, two egg (medium) chives, dill, cheddar cheese, iodized
    sea salt
Muffin, bran with whole wheat flour
Grapes, seedless, ½ cup
Coffee substitute, freshly brewed

Mid-Morning Snack

Cashews, raw, 6 nuts

Lunch

Turkey, light meat, baked, 4 oz
Asparagus spears, steamed, 4
Spring water

Mid-Afternoon Snack

Apple, winesap or green, medium

Dinner

Cottage cheese, 2 percent fat, one cup, flavored with caraway
    seeds, juice from one garlic clove and hint of iodized sea
    salt
Kiwi fruit
Chamomile tea

BASIC DIET
Daily Supplements

Vitamin A (from fish liver oils), 10,000 I.U.

Vitamin B-Complex, 50 mg of major B vitamins
(If your cholesterol is 220 or more, 500 mg of timed-release niacin, three times daily.)

Vitamin C, 1,000 mg, four times
(Reduce if you verge on diarrhea.)

Vitamin E (Alpha tocopherol), 200 I.U.

Calcium, oyster shell, 250 mg. four times
(This should contain 125 mg of Vitamin D.)

Magnesium, 250 mg, two times

Potassium, 550 mg

Selenium, 50 mcg

Zinc, 25 mg

GLA, 500 mg, 2 tabs three times

MAX-EPA, 1,000 mg, three times

Tryptophan, 667 mg

Make sure that your supplements contain no sugar, starch, artificial coloring or flavoring, or preservatives, any of which could cause food sensitivity or allergies.

CANDIDA ALBICANS VARIATION
Approximately 1,000 calories

Please note. Daily supplements follow the Fifth Day of this diet. No fruit is permitted because of its high sugar content. After three to six weeks, you may wish to try one fruit at a time and be alert for negative symptoms.

FIRST DAY

Breakfast

Halibut, baked or broiled, 4 oz
Toast, whole grain wheat, lightly buttered
Carrot, small, crunchy or grated
Taheebo tea

Mid-Morning Snack

Muffin, buckwheat flour with bran

Lunch

Eggs, 2 medium, soft or hardboiled
Green salad, Romaine lettuce, all you can eat, sunflower seed
     oil dressing, hint of garlic salt
Spring water

Mid-Afternoon Snack

Sunflower seeds, unsalted, 1 oz

Dinner

Baked sweet potato
Cabbage-carrot salad, grated, with unsweetened yogurt dressing
Taheebo tea

SECOND DAY

Breakfast

Oatmeal with soy milk
Green peas, raw, 2 oz
Toast, whole grain rye, lightly buttered
Taheebo tea

Mid-Morning Snack

Popcorn, air-popped, one cup, lightly buttered

Lunch

Lentil soup
Green salad, Romaine lettuce, alfalfa sprouts, olive oil dressing
Coffee substitute, freshly brewed

Mid-Afternoon Snack

Cauliflower, raw, four florets

Dinner

Irish potato, small, baked with skin, lightly buttered, dill, iodized
    sea salt
Green pepper, ½ cup cut in strips
Broccoli, cooked, ½ cup
Taheebo tea

THIRD DAY

Breakfast

Lamb shoulder chop, broiled, 4 oz
Asparagus spears, steamed, four medium size
Taheebo tea

Mid-Morning Snack

Pumpkin seeds, unsalted, 1 oz

Lunch

Salmon patty blended with freshly diced onions, broiled, 3 oz
Jicama slices, 3
Spring water

Mid-Afternoon Snack

Celery stick, medium, with almond butter

Dinner

Green salad, butter lettuce, all you can eat with soy oil dressing
Snap, green beans, steamed, 3 oz
Sweet corn, small ear, lightly buttered, touch of iodized sea salt
Taheebo tea

FOURTH DAY

Breakfast

Veal chop, broiled, 3 oz
Muffin, oat bran
Yellow squash, baked, 1 cup
Taheebo tea

Mid-Morning Snack

Cashew nuts, unsalted, 14 large

Lunch

Tuna salad with Boston lettuce (3 oz tuna). Safflower oil dressing
with hint of iodized sea salt
Spring water

Mid-Afternoon Snack

Pecans, large halves, 10

Dinner

Brown rice, short grain, cooked, beef broth flavoring added, ½
cup
Radishes, three
Brussels sprouts, three, sprinkled with freshly ground Parmesan
cheese
Taheebo tea

FIFTH DAY

You have the option of going back to the First Day or of using this in place of the First Day and then following through the cycle from the Second Day.

Breakfast

Chicken breast, baked, 4 oz
Red cabbage, raw, 3 oz wedge
Muffin, whole wheat and bran
Taheebo tea

Mid-Morning Snack

Pumpkin seeds, unsalted, 1 oz

Lunch

Omelet, two eggs, medium, chives, dill, iodized sea salt

Mid-Afternoon Snack

Brazil nuts, four

Dinner

Yam, small, baked, lightly buttered
Zucchini strips, ½ cup for dipping into low-fat, unsweetened
    yogurt and caraway seed dressing
Taheebo tea

CANDIDA ALBICANS DIET
Daily Supplements

Acidophilus (Lactobacillus acidophilus), liquid (unsweetened), two tablespoons before each meal or freeze-dried capsules, 3 before each meal

Garlic, liquid, odorless, six spurts from squeezable, plastic bottle, twice

GLA, 500 mg, 2 tabs three times

(Taheebo tea is included in the Candida Albicans Diet)

Vitamin A (from fish liver oils), 10,000 I.U.

Vitamin B-complex, 50 mg of major B vitamins (If your cholesterol is 220 or more, 500 mg of timed-release niacin, three times daily.)

Vitamin C, 1,000 mg, four times. Reduce if on verge of diarrhea.

Vitamin E (Alpha tocopherol), 200 I.U.

Calcium, oyster shell, 250 mg, four times (should also contain 125 mg of vitamin D)

Magnesium, 250 mg, two times

Potassium, 55 mg

Selenium, 50 mcg

Zinc, 25 mg

MAX-EPA, 1,000 mg, three times

Tryptophan, 667 mg

Make sure your supplements contain no sugar, starch, artificial coloring or flavoring, or preservatives, any of which could cause food sensitivity or allergies.

APPENDIX

Often I am asked what should be done clinically to rule out all health conditions discussed in this book as major unsuspected causes of your overweight.

My advice is to start with the best medical history and physical exam you can get. Then I recommend the following tests, particularly for new patients.

1. SMAC-20 chemistry panel, a fairly routine blood exam that reads cholesterol and triglyceride levels, liver and kidney function, and blood levels of electrolytes: sodium, potassium, and chloride.

2. Complete blood count with differential.

3. Thyroid function tests: T3, T4, FT1, YDH, T3R1A, antithyroid antibodies, TB11, Ts1. See Chapter two for more detail.

4. Glycohemoglobin, a relatively new blood test that measures the glucose levels inside your cells. This is an extremely sensitive indicator of how your body handles sugar, a key measurement to help you lose weight.

5. Magnesium level.

6. Urinalysis.

7. 12 lead electrocardiogram.

8. Serum cortisol level, a sensitive indicator of adrenal function.

9. Candida albicans yeast antibody studies, when indicated.

10. Epstein-Barr viral antibody studies, when indicated.

11. Blood antibody studies for specific food allergies: IGg and IGe.

Nutritionally, my patients are asked to:

1. Keep a dietary diary.

2. Complete a hair mineral analysis test to rule out toxic metal accumulations. Despite what you may have heard to the contrary, hair analysis is the best and cheapest screening test around for toxic metals.

3. Computerized Nutritional Evaluation.

4. Life-style and Stress Evaluation Test.

5. Blood vitamin and mineral levels.

If these tests are miraculously all negative, I would refer you to other physician specialists for further evaluation.

The main thing to remember when you're hurting, confused, and visiting a new doctor is not to think you're suffering from some rare ailment. You probably aren't. An old saying drummed into our heads in medical school was this:

"If you hear hoofbeats outside the window, don't expect to see a zebra."

The overwhelming majority of my patients who are chronically ill and overweight are not suffering from some exotic disease. Rather, they turn out to have one of the common but often unsuspected conditions we discuss in this book.

Therefore, it is best to have these easy-to-obtain, relatively inexpensive tests done before submitting to more exotic tests, unless there's a life-threatening emergency.

The advantages of regular exercise include:

1. Increased weight loss (what this book is all about)

2. Increased vitality

3. Curbed appetite

4. Relief of tension
5. Improvement in self-image and self-esteem
6. Increased mental alertness and productivity
7. Increased longevity

Most people are aware of the importance of exercise but do not follow a regular exercise routine because they feel it's too time-consuming or may require expensive equipment.

I've recently discovered what I consider to be the best home exerciser I've ever seen. It's called the *Tiger Band*.

The *Tiger Band* weighs less than a pound and is completely portable. It allows you to build strength while using a complete range of motion. In addition, it provides a complete aerobic workout as it increases flexibility. Anyone can use the *Tiger Band*—it is easily adaptable for men and women of any size or strength.

The *Tiger Band* exercise system retails for under $30 and comes with an illustrated wall chart that outlines suggested exercise programs easily performed at home. The system has been used for years, and is endorsed by hundreds of athletes and Olympic performers.

Further information on the *Tiger Band* system can be obtained by sending a self-addressed, stamped, business envelope to:

Tiger Band
P.O. Box 1549
LaFayette, CA 94549-1549

GLOSSARY

Preface

Allopathy: A term applied to that system of therapy in which diseases are treated by producing a condition incompatible with or antagonistic to the condition to be cured or alleviated. Example: the drug penicillin is used to treat a strep throat.

Amphetamine: A class of drugs used to stimulate the central nervous system, increase blood pressure, decrease appetite, and reduce nasal congestion.

Biochemical: The chemistry of living organisms.

Clinical effects of vitamin C: The physiological effects of vitamin C to help the body successfully kill viruses of all types; the ability of vitamin C to naturally aid the body in eliminating systemic poisons.

Clinical nutrition: The diagnosis and optimal correction of nutrient imbalances in an individual. Usually done by either a doctor specializing in nutrition or by nutritionists and dieticians who are specially trained.

Double-blind study: The study of the effects of a specific agent in which neither the administrator nor the recipient knows at the time of administration whether the active or inert substance is given.

F.D.A.: U.S. Food and Drug Administration.

Hodgkin's Disease: A malignant cancer of the lymph nodes and spleen.

Hypochondriasis: Severe anxiety about one's health, often associated with numerous and varying symptoms that cannot be attributed to organic disease.

I.V.: Intravenous.

Noninvasive: No penetration of the skin or body cavities, either in the diagnosis or the treatment of a bodily condition. Example: X-ray diagnosis is noninvasive. Surgery is invasive.

Organic: 1) Pertaining to an organ or organs; 2) Pertaining to or cultivated by the use of animal or vegetable fertilizers rather than synthetic chemicals.

Syndrome: A set of symptoms that occur together.

Chapter 1

Allergen: A substance capable of causing an allergy. An allergen may be a protein or non-protein.

Amino acid: The nutritional building block of proteins.

Assimilation: The transformation of food into living tissue.

Candida albicans: A fungus commonly found in the human body; its overgrowth can cause a variety of infections.

Clinical ecologist: A physician who specializes in the diagnosis and treatment of food and environmental allergies and/or sensitivities.

Endorphin: Any of a group of proteins with potent analgesic properties that occur naturally in the brain.

Folic acid: A member of the vitamin B complex.

Hypoglycemia: Low blood sugar.

Hypothyroid: An underactive thyroid.

Niacinamide: A member of the vitamin B family derived from niacin (vitamin B3). It occurs naturally in the body.

Pantotheninc acid, biotin, choline, inositol, PaBA: All vitamin B complex vitamins.

Subclinical: Without clinical manifestations, such as in the early stages of a disease.

Thyroid gland: The largest endocrine (ductless) gland in the human body, whose hormones act as a carburetor for every cell from our hair follicles to our toenails.

Chapter 2

Anemia: A reduction below normal in the number of red blood cells, or in the quantity of the cellular protein hemoglobin (which is responsible for binding oxygen and carrying it to the tissues), or a reduction in red blood cell volume (caused either by bleeding or by destruction of the blood cells by disease).

Antimicrosomal antithyroglobulin: Specific proteins found in the blood of people with autoimmune thyroiditis.

Arteriosclerosis: Hardening of the arteries.

Cholesterol: A fatlike substance found in animal fats and oil; also manufactured by the body.

Complex carbohydrate: Carbohydrate found in starchy vegetables, grains, and cereals.

Contractility: Capacity for becoming short in response to a suitable stimulus.

Desiccated: Freed from connective tissue and fat, dried, and powdered.

DNA: Deoxyribonucleic acid, the carrier of genetic information for all organisms except certain viruses.

Endocrinologist: Physician who specializes in the diagnosis and treatment of glandular disorders.

Estrogen: One of the female sex hormones produced by the ovaries.

Goiter belt: A geographical area with an unusually large number of people suffering with enlargement of the thyroid gland, causing a swelling in the front part of the neck. The condition usually is caused by a chronic iodine deficiency.

HAIT: Hashimoto's Auto Immune Thyroiditis.

Immunoglobulin: An animal protein endowed with known antibody activity.

Prednisone: An anti-inflammatory hormone produced by the adrenal glands.

RDA: Recommended daily allowance.

RNA: Ribonucleic acid, a chemical that transmits information from DNA to the protein-forming system of the cell.

Thiocyanide: A molecule containing the toxic metal cyanide.

Thyrotropus: A pituitary gland hormone that stimulates the thyroid gland.

Chapter 3

Gastrointestinal: Pertaining to the stomach or the intestines.

GLA: Gamma linoleic acid. A nutritional breakdown product of essential fats, essential for life and good health.

Lactobacillus: A strain of usually friendly bacteria found in the digestive system.

Myriad: Many.

Precipitius: A specific type of antibody.

Chapter 4

Adrenaline, cortesol: Hormones produced by the adrenal gland.
Bile: A fluid manufactured by the liver, concentrated by the gall bladder, and poured into the small intestine. Bile salts play an essential role in fat digestion and absorption.
Blood albumin: One of the major blood proteins.
Diabetes: A general term referring to disorders characterized by excess urine excretion.
Glucose: A sugar that provides energy for every cell in the body.
Glycogen: The form of glucose stored in the liver and muscles.
Histamine: A chemical compound found in certain blood cells necessary for the proper functioning of the circulatory system, lungs, and stomach. It also plays a major role in causing certain allergic reactions.
Hypercholesterolemia: Abnormally high elevation of blood cholesterol.
Insulin: The blood-lowering hormone produced by the pancreas.
Insulinase: A bodily protein known as an enzyme, which destroys or inactivates insulin.
Lecithin: Fatty molecules found in animal tissues such as nerves, semen, liver, egg yolk.
Metabolism: The sum of all physical and chemical processes by which living, organized substance is produced and maintained, also the transformation by which energy is made available for the uses of the organism.
Methionine: An essential amino acid.
Subclinical malnutrition: A condition resulting from inadequate consumption of essential nutrients. Sustained over a long period of time, this condition may lead to chronic degenerative disease.

Chapter 5

Dander: Small scales from the hair or feathers of animals, which may cause allergic reactions in sensitive individuals.
Dermatitis: Inflammation of the skin.
Eczema: A superficial skin inflammation.
Enzyme: An often essential protein capable of accelerating a biochemical reaction.
Immunology: The study of immunity or how the body responds to foreign substances; the biological recognition of self from not self.

Post-nasal drip: A condition characterized by a sinus drainage behind the nose and into the throat.

Chapter 6

ACTH: A pituitary hormone that stimulates the adrenal glands.
Adrenal cortex: The outer layer of the adrenal gland.
Adrenal medulla: The inner layers of the adrenal gland.
Gland: An organ specialized to produce materials not related to their ordinary metabolic needs.
Hormone: A chemical substance often produced by the glands, which helps regulate the activity of a certain organ.
Linoleic acid: An essential fatty acid.
Lymph gland: Specialized organs found throughout the body that play a key role in the immune system.
Pituitary gland: The master gland in the human body. Connected by a stalk to the brain.
Thymus gland: An organ located at the base of the neck that plays a role in the immune system.
Ulcerative colitis: A disease characterized by ulcers in certain areas of the large intestines.

Chapter 7

Atopic: Allergic.
Complete protein: A protein that contains all of the essential amino acids (that the body cannot manufacture).
Emphysema: A chronic lung disease often caused by heavy smoking, which results in an irreversible destruction of lung tissue.
Glomerulonephritis: An inflammation of the filtering units (glomerulii) of the kidney.
Hemolytic anemic: An anemia caused by the separation of the essential oxygen-carrying protein hemoglobin from the red blood cells.
Kaposi's Sarcoma: A lung tumor characteristically found in AIDS patients.
Macrophage: A large cell that ingests microorganisms, other cells, or foreign particles.
Proteinuria: The presence of protein in the urine, often associated with a kidney defect or disease.

Systemic Lupus Erythematosis: An autoimmune disease of the connective tissues mainly affecting middle-aged women, often characterized by skin eruptions, joint pains, and fever.

T Lymphocytes: Specific white blood cells manufactured by the immune system.

Chapter 8

Asthma: A chronic disease characterized by periodic breathlessness and wheezing due to spasms of the main air passages or bronchii. Often an allergic condition.

Betaine Hydrochloride: An organic form of hydrochloric acid.

Bronchitis: An inflammation of the main air passages or bronchii.

Cardiovascular: Pertaining to the heart or circulatory system.

Lipotropin: An agent that hastens the removal or decreases the deposit of fat in the body.

Pleurisy: An inflammation of the tissue that lines the lungs (pleura).

Chapter 9

Folic acid: A member of the vitamin B complex family.

Tryptophan: An essential amino acid.

Chapter 10

Adiposity: Pertaining to the deposit of fatty tissues.

Aortic dissection: A life-threatening partial rupture of the wall of the aorta.

Apnea: Cessation of breathing.

BMI: Basal metabolic index—A measurement of how much energy the body is producing at rest. Generally performed soon after awakening.

Chenodeoxycholic acid: The third most abundant acid in human bile.

Diabetagenic: Producing diabetes atherogenic, producing hardening of the arteries.

Diastolic: The dilation period of the heart. It coincides with the interval between the second and first heart sounds.

Dysfunction: Abnormality or impairment of the functioning of an organ.

Hyperinsulinemia: The abnormal production of insulin.

Hypertension: High blood pressure.

Ileal bypass: An intestinal operation sometimes performed on people who are severely overweight.

Ischemic: Deficiency of blood in a part due to a construction or actual obstruction of a blood vessel.

Lipoprotein: A combination of lipid (fat) and protein possessing the general property of a protein. Practically all the lipids of the blood are present as lipoprotein complex.

Morbid obesity: Gross overweight.

Myocardial infarction: The death of heart tissue; heart attack.

Preeclampsia: The condition in a pregnant woman prior to eclampsia, i.e., onset of convulsions and coma, associated with high blood pressure, fluid retention, and protein in the urine.

Toxins: Poisons.

Chapter 14

Catecholamine: A group of compounds whose action mimics the effects of impulses conveyed by the sympathetic nervous system. Such compounds include Dopamine and Norepinephrine.

Mitochondria: Principal sites in the cell for the manufacture of energy.

Chapter 17

Chelating agent: A chemical compound in which a metallic ion is captured and firmly bound into a ring within the chelating molecule. Chelating agents are used in metal poisonings.

REFERENCES

Chapter 2

1. Gerald S. Levey, "Hypothyroidism: A Treacherous Masquerader," *Acute Care Medicine* (May, 1984): 34–36.
2. Broda O. Barnes, M.D., and Lawrence Galton, *Hypothyroidism: the Unsuspected Illness* (New York: Crowell, 1976): 46.
3. Edward R. Pinckney, "The Accuracy and Significance of Medical Testing," *Archives of Internal Medicine* (March, 1983): 143:3, 512.
4. J. C. Scott, Jr., and Elizabeth Mussey, "Menstrual Patterns in Myxedema," *American Journal of Obstetrics and Gynecology* (1965): 90: 161.
5. Isobel W. Jennings, *Vitamins in Endocrine Metabolism* (Springfield, Ill.: Charles C. Thomas, 1970): 41.
6. *Medical Clinics of America* (1985): 1044.

Chapter 4

1. D. Diengott et al, *Endocrinology* (1959): 65, 602.
2. C. M. Leevy et al, *Archives of Internal Medicine* (1953): 92, 527.

Chapter 5

1. Interview with James Braly, M.D., by James F. Scheer.

Chapter 6

1. *Science News* (August 6, 1983): 124, 6: 84.
2. C. J. Tui, *Journal of Clinical Nutrition* (1953): 1, 232.
3. Ibid.
4. *The Complete Book of Vitamins* (Emmaus, Pa.: Rodale Press, 1977): 118.
5. Ibid.
6. W. A. Krehl, *American Journal of Clinical Nutrition* (1962): 11, 77.
7. A. F. Morgan et al, *Journal of Biological Chemistry* (1952): 195, 583.
8. *Complete Book of Vitamins* (Emmaus, Pa.: Rodale Press, 1977): 243.
9. B. L. Smolyanski, *Federation Proceedings* (1963): 22, T 1173.
10. *Nutrition Reviews* (1960): 18, 179.
11. L. S. Hurley, et al, *Journal of Biological Chemistry* (1952): 195, 583.
12. Ibid., H. J. Rosenkrantz (1956): 223, 47 and (1957): 224, 165.
13. William M. Jefferies, *Safe Uses of Cortisone* (Springfield, Ill.: Charles C. Thomas, Publisher, 1981): Preface, V.
14. Caroline B. Thomas, "Stamina: The Thread of Human Life," *Journal of Chronic Diseases* (July–August, 1981): 34: 41–44.

Chapter 7

1. Carl C. Pfeiffer, *Mental and Elemental Nutrients* (New Canaan, CT.: Keats Publishing, Inc., 1975): 316.
2. Ibid., 316.
3. Robert H. Garrison, Jr., and Elizabeth Somer, *The Nutrition Desk Reference* (New Canaan, CT.: Keats Publishing, Inc., 1985): 79.
4. Ibid., 175.
5. Ibid., 79.
6. *The Health Finder* (Emmaus, Pa.: Rodale Books, Inc., 1959): 485–486.
7. David W. Eggleston, "Effect of Dental Amalgam and Nickel Alloys on T-Lymphocytes: Preliminary Report," *The Journal of Prosthetic Dentistry* (May, 1984): Vol. 51, No. 5, 617–623.

Chapter 8

1. *1984–85 Yearbook of Nutritional Medicine* (New Canaan, CT.: Keats Publishing, Inc., 1985): 126.
2. Ibid., 126.
3. Ibid., 127.
4. Ibid., 127.
5. Ibid., 127.
6. Ibid., 232.
7. *The Complete Book of Vitamins* (Emmaus, Pa.: Rodale Press, 1977): 266.

Chapter 9

1. Joseph P. Hrachovec, *Keeping Young and Living Longer* (Los Angeles, CA.: Sherbourne Press, Inc., 1972): 64.
2. Ibid., 64.
3. Leonard Kotkin, *Eat, Think and Be Slender* (Los Angeles, CA: Wilshire Book Company, 1955): 40–43.
4. Richard B. Stuart and Barbara Davis, *Slim Chance in a Fat World*, (Champaign, Ill.: Research Press, 1972): 50, 51.
5. Ibid., 51.
6. Ibid., 51.
7. Ibid., 86.
8. Edward E. Abramson, *Behavioral Approaches to Weight Control* (New York, N.Y.: Springer Publishing Company, 1977): 8.
9. Ibid., 8.
10. Jean Mayer, *Overweight Causes, Costs & Control* (Englewood Cliffs, N.J.: Prentice-Hall. Inc., 1968): 94.
11. Ibid., 94.
12. Ibid., 94.
13. Mark Bricklin, *The Practical Encyclopedia of Natural Healing*, New, Revised Edition (Emmaus, Pa.: Rodale Press, 1983): 143.

Chapter 10

1. P. Bjorntorp, *Annals of Clinical Research* (1985): 17 (1), 39.
2. J. Bass and J. B. Freeman, *Adv. Surgery* (1984): 18: 55, 223.
3. *British Medical Journal* (May 12, 1984): 288 (6428), 1401–4.

4. *American Journal of Epidemiology* (April, 1984): 119: 4. 526–40.
5. *American Journal of Medicine* (December, 1984): 77 (6), 1077–82.
6. *Acta Medica Scandinavia* (1984): 216 (3), 277–285.
7. *Circulation* (March 7, 1985): 1 (3), 481–6.
8. *American Journal of Cardiology* (March 1, 1985): 2 (1), 85–91.
9. *Journal of Hypertension* (Feb, 1984): 2 (1), 85–91.
10. *Biomedical Pharmacotherapy* (1983): 37 (6), 251–8.
11. *Lancet* (June 1, 1985): 1 (8440), 1233–6.
12. *International Journal of Obesity* (1984): 8 (2), 138–40.
13. *Metabolism* (Mar, 1985): 34 (3), 227–36.
14. Robert H. Garrison, Jr., and Elizabeth Somer, *The Nutrition Desk Reference* (New Canaan, CT.: Keats Publishing, Inc., 1985): 143.
15. *Nutrition-Cancer* (1981): 2 (4), 237–40.
16. *American Journal of Epidemiology* (Aug, 1984): 120 (1), 244–50.
17. "Conference on Diabetes and Obesity," *The Sciences* (June, 1967): 7:1, 13–14.
18. *Journal of Experimental Medicine* (Dec, 1983): 141 Supplement, 142–6.
19. Ibid., 147–59
20. *American Journal of Clinical Nutrition* (April, 1985): 41 (4), 776–83.
21. *American Journal of Medicine* (Nov 30, 1983): 75 (5B) 32–40.
22. *Obstetrical-Gynecological Surgery* (Feb, 1985): 40 (2), 57–60.
23. *International Journal of Obesity* (1984): 8 (6). 681–8.
24. *Respiration* (1984): 45 (4) 321–6.
25. *American Journal of Cardiology* (Nov 1, 1984): 54 (8) 1887–91.
26. *Journal of the American Dietetic Association* (April, 1965): 85 (4), 483–4.

Chapter 12

1. Richard B. Stuart and Barbara Davis, *Slim Chance in a Fat World* (Champaign, Ill.: Research Press, 1972), 47.
2. Ibid., 47, 48.
3. Ibid., 48.
4. Ibid., 49.
5. Ibid., 49.

6. Ibid., 50.
7. Ibid., 50.

Chapter 13

1. Interview with Grant Gwinup by James F. Scheer.
2. Jean Mayer, *Overweight Causes, Cost and Control* (Englewood Cliffs, N.J.: Prentice-Hall, Inc., 1968): 72, 73.
3. Ibid., 73.
4. Ibid., 73, 74.
5. Ibid., 76, 77.
6. Ibid., 77.
7. Ibid., 71.
8. Ibid., 79.
9. Stephen E. Langer with James F. Scheer, *Solved: The Riddle of Illness* (New Canaan, CT.: Keats Publishing, Inc., 1984): 142.

Chapter 14

1. *Science 82* (Mar, 1982): 42.
2. *Your Health* (Mar 18, 1986): 16–18.
3. *Experientia* (Supplement) (1983): 44, 26–44.
4. Ibid., 44, 26–44.
5. Jean Mayer, *Overweight Causes, Cost and Control* (Englewood Cliffs, N.J.: Prentice Hall, Inc., 1968): 157.
6. *American Journal of Clinical Nutrition* (July, 1985): 42 (1), 83–94.
7. *Clinical Endocrinology* (Oxf) (Oct 21, 1984): (4), 357–67.
8. *Clinical Endocrinology-Metabolism* (Nov, 1984): 13 (3), 581–95.
9. Ibid.
10. *Aesthetic Plastic Surgery* (1984): 8 (1), 13–17.
11. Charles T. Kuntzelman, *Diet Free* (Emmaus, Pa.: Rodale Press, 1981): 285.

Chapter 15

1. Richard Passwater, *Supernutrition* (New York, N.Y.: The Dial Press, 1975): 23.

2. *Journal of the Louisiana State Medical Society* (1985): 137 (6): 35–8.

Chapter 16

1. Richard B. Stuart and Barbara Davis, *Slim Chance in a Fat World*, (Champaign, Ill.: Research Press, 1972): 25.
2. News Story, "Fad Diets Are Losers, Say Reese Doctors," Michael Reese Hospital and Medical Center, Oct. 14, 1977.
3. Ibid., 1.
4. Ibid., 2.
5. Ibid., 2.
6. Ibid., 3.
7. Ibid., 3.
8. Ibid., 4.
9. Ibid., 4.
10. Stuart and Davis, *Slim Chance in a Fat World* (Champaign, Ill.: Research Press, 1972): 89.
11. Jean Mayer, *Overweight Causes, Cost and Control* (Englewood Cliffs, N.J.: Prentice-Hall, Inc., 1968): 196.
12. "Fad Diets," *Postgraduate Medicine* (Jan, 1986): 79:1, 249–255.
13. "The Fructose Connection: Copper and Heart Disease," *Science News* (May 3, 1986): 129:18, 279.

Chapter 17

1. William A. Albrect, "Diseases vs. Deficiencies via the Soil," *Natural Food and Farming Digest* (1957): 106–109.
2. *The Yearbook of Agriculture, 1959* (Washington, D.C.: United States Department of Agriculture): 391–392.
3. Allan Cott, testimony before Select Committee on Nutrition and Human Needs of the United States Senate, June 22, 1977, from "Diet Related to Killer Diseases," (Washington, D.C., U.S. Government Printing Office, 1977): 268.
4. Ibid., 96.
5. Richard Passwater, *Supernutrition* (New York, N.Y.: The Dial Press, 1975): 18.
6. Stephen E. Langer with James F. Scheer, *Solved: The Riddle of*

Illness (New Canaan, CT.: Keats Publishing, Inc., 1984): 81–82.

7. Interview by James F. Scheer.

Chapter 18

1. *Bibliotecha Nutritio Dieta* (1985): (35) 111–121.
2. *International Journal of Obesity* (1979): 3 (3), 201–211.
3. *Metabolism* (Sep, 1984): 33 (9), 820–5.
4. Ibid., (Mar, 1985): 34 (3), 285–93.
5. *International Journal of Obesity* (1984, 8 Supplement): 79–84.
6. *Appetito* (Mar, 1984): 6 (1), 25–40.
7. *International Journal of Obesity* (1982): 6 (1), 43–52.
8. Mark Bricklin, *The Practical Encyclopedia of Natural Healing* (Emmaus, Pa.: Rodale Press, 1983): 186–187.
9. Jeffrey Bland, *Medical Applications of Clinical Nutrition* (New Canaan, CT.: Keats Publishing, Inc., 1983): 108.
10. Interview by James F. Scheer.

Chapter 19

1. "High Fiber Diet Has Its Drawbacks," *Los Angeles Times* (June 28, 1985).
2. *Postgraduate Medicine Journal* (1984): 60 supplement 3, 50–55.
3. Mark Bricklin, *The Practical Encyclopedia of Natural Healing* (Emmaus, Pa.: Rodale Press, 1983): 210.
4. *Acta Paediatrica-Hungary* (1985): 26 (1), 75–7.
5. *Bibliotecha Nutritio Dieta* (1985): (35), 111–127.
6. News Story, U.S. Dept. of Agriculture, Washington, D.C., May 23, 1983.
7. *Yearbook of Nutritional Medicine* (New Canaan, CT.: Keats Publishing, Inc., 1985): 290.
8. Lawrence Power, *Los Angeles Times* (Jan 14, 1979): Part IV, 4.
9. *British Journal of Nutrition* (July, 1984): 52 (1), 97–105.

Chapter 20

1. *International Journal of Obesity* (1984): 8 (4), 289–93.
2. *Journal of Lipid Research* 4 (1963): 279–288.

3. Brian Leibovitz, *Carnitine, The Vitamin B_T Phenomenon* (New York, N.Y.: Dell Publishing Co., 1984): 29.
4. Ibid., 108.
5. Ibid., 110.
6. David F. Horrobin, "The Role of Essential Fatty Acids and Evening Primrose Oil in the Regulation of Body Weight and Diabetes Mellitus," lecture to annual meeting of the American Society of Bariatric Physicians, Las Vegas, Nevada, October 15, 1981.
7. Ibid.
8. Ibid.

INDEX